"It is a great pleasure to endorse this important book by Dr. Michal Nissim. Her rich theoretical knowledge and clinical experience offer readers deep insights into hydrotherapy within disability paradigms. The holistic model presented is timely and essential, offering a comprehensive framework for diverse therapeutic practices."

Professor Navah Ratzon, *Tel Aviv University, Israel*

"This book is a unique contribution to the field of hydrotherapy and aquatic exercise, uniting lived experience with theoretical depth. Through an innovative four-dimensional model, it promotes holistic well-being and critical reflection. By integrating practical knowledge with academic rigour, it empowers professionals to enhance their therapeutic work and deepen inclusion."

Professor Yeshayahu (Shayke) Hutzler, *Professor of Adapted Physical Activity and Rehabilitation, Head of the Centre for Innovation and Entrepreneurship, Levinsky-Wingate Academic Center; Former President of IFAPA (International Federation of Adapted Physical Activity), Israel*

Inclusive Hydrotherapy

This text provides a comprehensive introduction to using hydrotherapy as a means of promoting autonomy and social inclusion for individuals with disabilities.

Reflecting the global transition from predominantly medical models of disability towards more inclusive and empowering approaches, the book presents the Four-Dimensional Model of Hydrotherapy – a conceptual framework that integrates physical functioning, sensory experience, positive identity development, and long-term well-being. With an evidence-based approach throughout, and informed by key hydrotherapy principles, the book synthesises current research across disability studies, rehabilitation sciences, and inclusive education. Structured case studies and applied examples illustrate how hydrotherapy can address challenges such as accessibility, staff training, and communication barriers, ensuring that interventions remain responsive across a range of settings.

This book will be of particular interest to allied health professionals working in physiotherapy, occupational therapy, speech and language therapy, and beyond. By bridging theory and practice, it provides a valuable resource for delivering inclusive, person-centred hydrotherapy aligned with contemporary disability rights frameworks.

Michal Nissim is Head of the Special Education Department at David Yellin College of Education, where she founded and leads the Hydrotherapy and Rehabilitation Swimming Programme. She holds a PhD in Special Education, with a research focus on aquatic motor interventions across the lifespan. She completed postdoctoral fellowships in neuroscience and occupational therapy. Nissim's work promotes inclusive, person-centred hydrotherapy practices that foster autonomy, participation, and well-being in diverse therapeutic and educational contexts.

Inclusive Hydrotherapy

A Guide to Interventions for Individuals with Disabilities

MICHAL NISSIM

Routledge
Taylor & Francis Group

LONDON AND NEW YORK

Cover design image: Getty Images

First published 2026
by Routledge
4 Park Square, Milton Park, Abingdon, Oxon OX14 4RN

and by Routledge
605 Third Avenue, New York, NY 10158

Routledge is an imprint of the Taylor & Francis Group, an informa business

© 2026 Michal Nissim

British Library Cataloguing-in-Publication Data
A catalogue record for this book is available from the British Library

ISBN: 978-1-041-11380-5 (hbk)
ISBN: 978-1-041-11379-9 (pbk)
ISBN: 978-1-003-65970-9 (ebk)

DOI: 10.4324/9781003659709

Typeset in Vectora LH
by SPi Technologies India Pvt Ltd (Straive)

To Jonathan, my partner in heart and mind,
and to our children: Yair, Ayala, and Beeri –
whose love, patience, and quiet strength carried me
across waters known and unknown.

To my parents, Rivka and Ze'ev Berenstin,
and to Yossi and Dina Nissim, my parents-in-law,
for their steady presence and boundless
encouragement.

To the therapists, swimmers, and individuals I have
met in the water,
and to the scholars whose words and wisdom
guided my steps.
Thank you for accompanying me, both afloat and on
firm ground.

Contents

Tables

Introduction

As the field of rehabilitation sciences continues to evolve, hydrotherapy is increasingly recognised not merely as a biomechanical intervention, but as a therapeutic space that fosters empowerment, participation, and inclusion. This shift raises a critical question: how can hydrotherapy combine a strong evidence-based foundation with responsiveness to the personal, diverse, and changing needs of the individuals who take part in it?

Hydrotherapy, also known as aquatic therapy, is a therapeutic approach that draws on the distinctive physical properties of water, such as buoyancy, hydrostatic pressure, thermal conductivity, and density, to support rehabilitation, promote neuromuscular recovery, and enhance overall well-being (Becker, 2009; Becker, 2020; Mooventhan & Nivethitha, 2014; Nissim et al., 2020; Nissim et al., 2024; Torres-Ronda & i del Alcázar, 2014). Traditionally, hydrotherapy has been grounded in biomechanical rehabilitation, focusing on supporting neuromuscular, cardiovascular, and respiratory function through aquatic-based interventions (Brody & Geigle, 2009; Cole & Becker, 2004). However, contemporary research and practice reveal a more holistic and multi-dimensional perspective, one that situates hydrotherapy not only as a means of physical rehabilitation but also as a vehicle for fostering social participation, self-determination, and the development of affirmative identity (Shariat et al., 2024; Shelef, 2010).

To fully appreciate the role of hydrotherapy within contemporary rehabilitation, it is necessary to situate it within the broader global context of disability and access to care. Disability affects a substantial, and growing, segment of the global population. Recent estimates suggest that approximately 13% of adults aged 15 and over in low- and middle-income countries experience functional difficulties, while household-level prevalence reaches a median of 28% (Mitra et al., 2023). Global analyses report national prevalence rates ranging from 11% to over 32%, with a

DOI: 10.4324/9781003659709-1

median of 21% across 15 countries representing diverse geographic and socio-economic contexts (Hanass-Hancock et al., 2023). Additionally, more than 2.4 billion people are expected to require rehabilitation services at some point in their lives, reflecting trends in population ageing and the rising burden of non-communicable diseases (Sabariego et al., 2022).

The economic and social implications of disability are wide-reaching. In addition to the challenges faced by individuals, families often encounter increased caregiving responsibilities, reduced income, and restricted access to essential services. At the societal level, exclusion from education and employment contributes to lost productivity and higher public expenditure. For example, while remote work has improved employment outcomes for some persons with disabilities, substantial disparities persist in wages and long-term job security (Bloom et al., 2024). Without inclusive labour policies and sustained investment in support systems, these inequities risk becoming further entrenched (Çelikay, 2023).

Health, education, and social care systems are under growing pressure to respond to the increasing demand for inclusive and effective rehabilitation services. Despite international commitments, such as the United Nations Convention on the Rights of Persons with Disabilities (CRPD) and the World Health Organization (WHO) Rehabilitation 2030 initiative, access to rehabilitation remains limited in many countries (Seijas et al., 2023). This lack of access contributes to prolonged hospital stays, diminished functional recovery, and restricted opportunities for social participation. Fragmented, under-resourced services place a disproportionate burden on individuals and families, especially in low-resource contexts, further exacerbating health and social inequities (McCusker et al., 2023).

In this context, hydrotherapy emerges as a vital component of comprehensive rehabilitation (Cole & Becker, 2004). Aquatic environments provide distinctive therapeutic advantages, they support movement, reduce joint loading, and enhance sensory processing (Carroll et al., 2020). A growing body of evidence demonstrates their effectiveness in improving balance, mobility, and neuromotor control in conditions such as Parkinson's disease and Muscular Dystrophy (Carroll et al., 2020; Israel, 2018). Moreover, qualitative research underscores the emotional and social significance of hydrotherapy. Participants describe these experiences as empowering and enjoyable, highlighting their role in facilitating meaningful activity and inclusive participation (Jackman et al., 2024).

Accordingly, hydrotherapy should not be regarded merely as a supplementary intervention, but also as a core component of inclusive, person-centred rehabilitation. Its capacity to improve health outcomes, promote autonomy, and reduce long-term dependency positions it as both a clinical priority and a social imperative within contemporary disability-responsive care.

At the centre of this book is the Four-Dimensional Model of Hydrotherapy, an integrative framework developed to expand hydrotherapy practice beyond its traditional biomedical focus. Grounded in principles from disability studies (Oliver, 2018; Shakespeare, 2015; Goodley, 2013), the International Classification of Functioning, Disability and Health (ICF) (WHO, 2001), and inclusive rehabilitation (Mpofu et al., 2010), the model foregrounds lived experience, and the socio-relational context of individuals participating in hydrotherapy.

The model comprises four interconnected dimensions, each contributing to a comprehensive, person-centred understanding of hydrotherapy:

1. Body Functioning & Sensory Experience- Addresses how water affects movement, balance, pain modulation, and sensory processing. It emphasises the role of the aquatic environment in supporting neuromuscular functioning and sensory integration, while recognising individual variability in physical and sensory responses (Becker, 2009; Torres-Ronda & i del Alcázar, 2014).
2. Affirmative Identity & Self-Determination- Explores how aquatic movement can foster self-efficacy, autonomy, emotional resilience, and self-expression. This dimension positions hydrotherapy as a space for identity development and empowerment, challenging deficit-based assumptions and promoting personal agency. It also recognises the importance of shared decision-making and communicative agency, emphasising that individuals should actively participate in shaping their rehabilitation process and advocating for their own needs (Shelef, 2010; Swain & French, 2000; Shakespeare, 2015).
3. Social Belonging & Inclusion- Examines the potential of hydrotherapy settings to promote equity, accessibility, and social connection. It calls for socially engaging, inclusive environments that reduce isolation and affirm a sense of belonging and community membership (Allen et al., 2022; Booth et al., 2002; Garcia et al., 2012; Shariat et al., 2024).
4. Holistic Well-Being & Long-Term Impact- Considers how hydrotherapy contributes not only to immediate rehabilitation goals but also to emotional resilience, life satisfaction, and sustained participation in meaningful daily activities (Mooventhan & Nivethitha, 2014).

Together, these dimensions support a shift towards a more inclusive, affirming, and context-responsive approach to hydrotherapy. The chapters that follow illustrate how the Four-Dimensional Model of Hydrotherapy can be applied across a range of techniques, populations, and settings, embedding hydrotherapy within a values-based framework that foregrounds dignity, equity, and relational connection.

This model integrates established aquatic rehabilitation principles (Cole & Becker, 2004) with critical insights from disability studies and social inclusion research (Darling, 2003; Linton, 1998; Swain & French, 2000), offering a conceptual shift away from traditional biomedical approaches. By bridging theory and practice, the model equips clinicians, educators, and researchers with a flexible framework for assessment, planning, and evaluation, adaptable across diverse contexts and responsive to personal goals.

One of the central challenges in hydrotherapy today lies in bridging the gap between research and practice. Inconsistent methodologies, assessment tools, and professional language across disciplines often hinder knowledge translation and collaborative development.

Among previous efforts to address this gap, ICF has played a particularly influential role. Adopted globally as a biopsychosocial framework, the ICF integrates medical and social perspectives on health and disability (WHO, 2001). The ICF and its adaptations, such as the ICF-CY (Children and Youth version), offer a structured approach to assessing body functions, activity limitations, and participation barriers, and provide a common language for planning and evaluating hydrotherapy interventions (Hadar-Frumer et al., 2023).

While the ICF effectively captures physical, environmental, and social interactions, it does not fully reflect the experiential and identity-based dimensions of rehabilitation. In particular, it offers limited guidance on how therapeutic processes, such as hydrotherapy, can foster empowerment, self-determination, and the development of a positive disability identity.

The Four-Dimensional Model of Hydrotherapy responds to this gap. Grounded in inclusive principles, the model offers a structured yet flexible framework that supports autonomy and participation. It lays the groundwork for practical application across diverse clinical and educational settings.

This practical application is illustrated through a series of structured case studies, each presented in accordance with the internationally recognised CARE (CAse REport) guidelines (Riley et al., 2017), ensuring methodological rigour and transparency. By integrating functional, psychological, social, and identity-based dimensions, the model supports inclusive, empowerment-oriented interventions that are both evidence-based and person-centred, enhancing clinical outcomes and supporting long-term well-being.

This book not only introduces the Four-Dimensional Model of Hydrotherapy, but also critically explores how this framework can be used to analyse and interpret established hydrotherapy techniques, such as the Halliwick Concept, the Bad Ragaz Ring Method (BRRM), Ai Chi, AquaStretch, and other widely recognised hydrotherapy practices. By applying the model as an interpretive lens, the book offers a structured analysis that acknowledges the distinct contributions of these techniques, while illustrating how a multidimensional perspective can deepen understanding and enhance inclusive rehabilitation practice. The model's four dimensions function not only as conceptual pillars, but also as analytical tools for examining the complex and layered impact of hydrotherapy. The following sections expand on each dimension in greater detail, drawing on empirical research, clinical insight, and established aquatic practices to explore their practical significance within inclusive therapeutic contexts.

In addition to its conceptual and clinical contributions, the Four-Dimensional Model of Hydrotherapy also offers international relevance. Its emphasis on shared professional language, theoretical coherence, and contextual adaptability enables implementation across diverse healthcare systems and institutional settings. This balance, standardised in principle yet flexible in practice, supports practitioners, educators, and researchers in developing inclusive hydrotherapy services that are responsive to both global standards and local needs.

Beyond its theoretical and conceptual contributions, this book serves as a practical and pedagogical resource, supporting hydrotherapy professionals, educators, service providers, and policy-makers in implementing inclusive, rights-based rehabilitation practices. It equips practitioners with both theoretical insight and applied tools to deliver person-centred, empowerment-oriented interventions across diverse populations and settings. In both clinical and educational contexts, the book offers future professionals a structured framework for applying evidence-based approaches that reflect the principles of inclusion and participation.

The model aligns with international disability rights frameworks, most notably the United Nations CRPD (United Nations, 2006), by advocating for equitable access to rehabilitation and community-based therapeutic services. Furthermore, it addresses real-world barriers, such as limited infrastructure and accessibility constraints, by offering adaptable, context-sensitive solutions that can be tailored to local needs and resources (Mulligan & Polkinghorne, 2013; Nissim et al., 2021).

This book offers hydrotherapy practitioners practical guidance for implementing the Four-Dimensional Model of Hydrotherapy, ensuring that interventions are person-centred, responsive to individual goals, and designed to maximise therapeutic potential while fostering inclusion and personal agency. For researchers, it provides a theoretical foundation for structured, evidence-based evaluation of hydrotherapy's effects, while integrating the lived experiences and voices of those who engage in aquatic therapy.

As hydrotherapy continues to evolve, this book invites practitioners, researchers, educators, and service providers to adopt a holistic, collaborative, and rights-based approach. More than a therapeutic method, the Four-Dimensional Model of Hydrotherapy challenges us to reimagine hydrotherapy not only as a means of restoring function, but as a relational space for empowerment, identity, and social change.

REFERENCES

Allen, K. A., Gray, D. L., Baumeister, R. F., & Leary, M. R. (2022). The need to belong: A deep dive into the origins, implications, and future of a foundational construct. *Educational Psychology Review*, *34*(2), 1133–1156.

Becker, B. E. (2009). Aquatic therapy: Scientific foundations and clinical rehabilitation applications. *PM&R*, *1*(9), 859–872.

Becker, B. E. (2020). Aquatic therapy in contemporary neurorehabilitation: An update. *PM&R*, *12*(12), 1251–1259.

Bloom, N., Dahl, G. B., & Rooth, D. O. (2024). *Work from Home and Disability Employment* (No. w32943). National Bureau of Economic Research.

Booth, T., Black-Hawkins, K., & Ainscow, M. (2002). *Guía para la Evaluación y Mejora de la Educación Inclusiva*. Madrid: Consorcio Universitario para la Educación Inclusiva.

Brody, L. T., & Geigle, P. R. (eds). (2009). *Aquatic Exercise for Rehabilitation and Training*. Human Kinetics.

Carroll, L. M., Morris, M. E., O'Connor, W. T., & Clifford, A. M. (2020). Is aquatic therapy optimally prescribed for Parkinson's disease? A systematic review and meta-analysis. *Journal of Parkinson's Disease*, *10*(1), 59–76.

Çelikay, F. (2023). Social spending and chronic unemployment: Evidence from OECD countries. *Review of Economics and Political Science*, *8*(2), 86–107.

Cole, A. J. & Becker, B. E. (2004). *Comprehensive Aquatic Therapy*. Butterworth Heinemann.

Darling, R. B. (2003). Toward a model of changing disability identities: A proposed typology and research agenda. *Disability & Society*, *18*(7), 881–895.

Garcia, J. M., da Silva, L. S., & Alves, A. L. (2012). The Halliwick Concept: Swimming instruction and therapy for individuals with disabilities. *Brazilian Journal of Physical Therapy*, *16*(2), 108–115.

Goodley, D. (2013). Dis/entangling critical disability studies. *Disability & Society*, *28*(5), 631–644.

Hadar-Frumer, M., Ten Napel, H., Yuste-Sánchez, M. J., & Rodríguez-Costa, I. (2023). The international classification of functioning, disability and health: Accuracy in aquatic activities reports among children with developmental delay. *Children*, *10*(5), 908.

Hanass-Hancock, J., Murthy, G. V. S., Palmer, M., Pinilla-Roncancio, M., Rivas Velarde, M., & Mitra, S. (2023). The disability data report 2023. *Disability Data Initiative*.

Israel, V. L. (2018). Aquatic assessment of motor skills in muscular dystrophy: A case study. *The Journal of Aquatic Physical Therapy*, *26*(1), 21–23.

Jackman, P. C., Cooke, S., George, T., Blackwell, J., & Middleton, G. (2024). Physical activity experiences of community-dwelling older adults with physical disabilities: A scoping review of qualitative research. *Disability and Rehabilitation*, *46*(16), 3564–3576.

Linton, S. (1998). *Claiming Disability: Knowledge and Identity*. NYU Press.

McCusker, P., Gillespie, L., Davidson, G., Vicary, S., & Stone, K. (2023). The United Nations convention on the rights of persons with disabilities and social work: Evidence for impact? *International Journal of Environmental Research and Public Health*, *20*(20), 6927.

Mitra, S., Yap, J., Hervé, J., & Chen, W. (2023). Inclusive statistics: A disaggregation of indicators by disability status and its implications for policy. *Global Social Policy*, *23*(1), 39–66.

Mooventhan, A., & Nivethitha, L. (2014). Scientific evidence-based effects of hydrotherapy on various systems of the body. *North American Journal of Medical Sciences*, *6*(5), 199.

Mpofu, E., Bishop, M., Hirschi, A., & Hawkins, T. (2010). Assessment of values. In E. Mpofu & T. Oakland (eds), *Rehabilitation and Health Assessment: Applying ICF Guidelines* (pp. 381–398). Springer Publishing Company.

Mulligan, H. F., & Polkinghorne, A. (2013). Inclusive hydrotherapy: Accessibility barriers and solutions. *International Journal of Aquatic Therapy*, *11*(2), 45–59.

Nissim, M., Ariel, N., & Alter, E. (2021). Practical applications of aquatic physical activity, swimming, and therapy for people with visual impairment or blindness. *Movement*, *13*(1). www.wincol.ac.il/publications/the_academic_college_at_wingate/bitnua/archive/2021_01/Prac.ical_Applications_of_Aquatic_Physical_Activity/

Nissim, M., Livny, A., Barmatz, C., Tsarfaty, G., Berner, Y., Sacher, Y., ... & Ratzon, N. Z. (2020). Effects of aquatic physical intervention on fall risk, working memory and hazard-perception as pedestrians in older people: A pilot trial. *BMC Geriatrics*, *20*, 1–12.

Nissim, M., Rottenberg, Y., Karniel, N., & Ratzon, N. Z. (2024). Effects of aquatic exercise program versus on-land exercise program on cancer-related fatigue, neuropathy, activity and participation, quality of life, and return to work for cancer patients: Study protocol for a randomized controlled trial. *BMC Complementary Medicine and Therapies*, *24*(1), 74.

Oliver, M. (2018). *Understanding Disability: From Theory to Practice*. Bloomsbury publishing.

Riley, D. S., Barber, M. S., Kienle, G. S., Aronson, J. K., von Schoen-Angerer, T., Tugwell, P., ... & Gagnier, J. J. (2017). CARE guidelines for case reports: Explanation and elaboration document. *Journal of Clinical Epidemiology*, *89*, 218–235.

Sabariego, C., Fellinghauer, C., Lee, L., Kamenov, K., Posarac, A., Bickenbach, J., ... & Cieza, A. (2022). Generating comprehensive functioning and disability data worldwide: Development process, data analyses strategy and reliability of the WHO and World Bank Model Disability Survey. *Archives of Public Health*, *80*(1), 6.

Seijas, V., Kiekens, C., & Gimigliano, F. (2023). Advancing the world health assembly's landmark resolution on strengthening rehabilitation in health systems: Unlocking the future of rehabilitation. *European Journal of Physical and Rehabilitation Medicine*, *59*(4), 447.

Shakespeare, T. (2015). Disability Research Today. London: Routledge.

Shariat, A., Najafabadi, M. G., Dos Santos, I. K., Anastasio, A. T., Milajerdi, H. R., Hassanzadeh, G., & Nouri, E. (2024). The effectiveness of aquatic therapy on motor and social skill as well as executive function in children with neurodevelopmental disorder: A systematic review and meta-analysis. Archives of Physical Medicine and Rehabilitation, 105(5), 1000–1007.

Shelef, A. N. (2010). Enhancing quality of life through aquatics therapy: Effectiveness of adaptation of seating posture loading in a partially immersed aquatics therapy approach for the improved functioning and perceived competence of children with cerebral palsy, as reflected in their quality of life: A multiple case study (Doctoral dissertation, Anglia Ruskin Research Online (ARRO)). Anglia Ruskin University.

Swain, J., & French, S. (2000). Towards an affirmation model of disability. *Disability & Society*, *15*(4), 569–582.

Torres-Ronda, L., & i del Alcázar, X. S. (2014). The properties of water and their applications for training. *Journal of Human Kinetics*, *44*, 237.

United Nations. (2006). *Convention on the Rights of Persons with Disabilities*. www.un.org/development/desa/disabilities/convention-on-the-rights-of-persons-with-disabilities.html

World Health Organization. (2001). *International Classification of Functioning, Disability and Health (ICF)*. World Health Organization.

Part I
Foundations
Hydrotherapy and Disability Paradigms

Chapter 1
Hydrotherapy and its Physiological Foundations

A HISTORICAL AND CONTEMPORARY OVERVIEW OF HYDROTHERAPY

Hydrotherapy, also referred to as aquatic therapy, aquatic rehabilitation, or water therapy, is the therapeutic use of water to promote health, rehabilitation, and overall well-being (Cole & Becker, 2004). Rooted in a long-standing tradition that spans centuries, hydrotherapy has deep historical origins that highlight the enduring relationship between humanity and water as a healing element. Ancient civilisations, most notably the Greeks and Romans, recognised the multifaceted therapeutic properties of water, incorporating it into daily life and formal medical practices (van Tubergen & van der Linden, 2002). Hippocrates (460–370 BC), often regarded as the father of modern medicine, advocated bathing in natural spring waters as a treatment for a variety of health conditions, and emphasised the holistic role of water immersion in supporting physical, emotional, and general well-being (Bender et al., 2002). His teachings laid a foundation that would profoundly influence medical thought for centuries.

The Romans, building on Greek traditions, institutionalised the practice by developing elaborate public thermal bath complexes, which served not only as places for healing but also as important social and cultural centres (Ring, 1996; Becker, 2009). These grand bathhouses symbolised an integrated approach to health that combined hygiene, physical therapy, social interaction, and relaxation. However, following the collapse of the Roman Empire in 476 CE, the practice of public bathing significantly declined. Religious shifts, coupled with increasing fears about disease transmission, particularly during outbreaks of plague, leprosy, and other infectious diseases, led to widespread closures of public baths and a retreat from communal water-based practices (van Tubergen & van der Linden, 2002; Cole & Becker, 2004).

DOI: 10.4324/9781003659709-3

Despite this historical regression, the Renaissance period of the 16th century marked a vibrant resurgence of interest in hydrotherapy. Italian physicians, inspired by the renewed study of classical Greek and Roman medical texts, began systematically re-examining the benefits of thermal water treatments. Their scholarly efforts identified over 78 specific health conditions that could potentially be alleviated through therapeutic immersion, ranging from musculoskeletal disorders to conditions affecting emotional well-being (van Tubergen & van der Linden, 2002). This revival set the stage for the more formalised development of hydrotherapy as a recognised and evidence-based modality within modern rehabilitation sciences.

Beyond Europe, numerous cultures embraced hydrotherapy for its healing potential. Throughout history, societies across Asia, Africa, and the Americas recognised the therapeutic properties of water and developed diverse traditions centred on its use for health and wellness. Chinese health practitioners promoted the use of warm springs, believing in water's ability to absorb and radiate heat for therapeutic purposes (Fields, 1950). This practice was often integrated into broader systems of medicine that emphasised balance, energy flow, and the harmonisation of bodily elements. Similarly, Indian and Egyptian civilisations integrated hydrotherapy into their health practices, utilising soaking waters for relaxation, cleansing, and fever reduction (Irion, 1997; Burns & Burns, 1997; De Vierville, 1997). These cultures viewed water not merely as a means of physical cleansing, but as a medium for spiritual purification and renewal, reflecting the interconnectedness of body, mind, and spirit in their healing philosophies. Indigenous communities in North America also recognised the benefits of mineral springs, incorporating them into traditional healing practices (Cole & Becker, 2004). Among these communities, mineral springs were revered as sacred spaces, often associated with ceremonial practices that reinforced social bonds and communal identity alongside physical healing.

The 20th century marked substantial advancements in the field of hydrotherapy. As medical science evolved, hydrotherapy began to transition from a traditional healing art into a more formalised and systematically studied therapeutic discipline. In the early 1900s, the practice began to incorporate structured movement through hydrogymnastics, considered one of the earliest formal approaches to aquatic therapy (Brody & Geigle, 2009). This method introduced targeted exercises in water to enhance strength, flexibility, and cardiovascular endurance, laying the groundwork for modern aquatic rehabilitation protocols. By the late 20th century, hydrotherapy had gained increased professional recognition, supported by empirical evidence demonstrating its effectiveness in facilitating recovery from injury and enhancing functional mobility (Cole & Becker, 2004).

Studies conducted during this period provided crucial validation for hydrotherapy's physiological benefits, promoting its integration into multidisciplinary rehabilitation programmes and its acceptance within mainstream medical and allied health practices.

PHYSICAL PROPERTIES OF WATER

Hydrotherapy's therapeutic benefits stem from the unique physical properties of water, which distinguish it from land-based therapy. These properties form the scientific foundation of hydrotherapy's clinical applications and are essential to understanding the mechanisms through which aquatic interventions achieve their effects. These properties include buoyancy, hydrostatic pressure, viscosity, temperature effects, and hydrodynamics, each contributing to the physiological effects that support rehabilitation and exercise (Becker, 2009; Cole & Becker, 2004). Each of these principles interacts dynamically with the human body, offering therapeutic advantages that cannot be replicated in terrestrial environments. Understanding these principles is fundamental to optimising hydrotherapy interventions for diverse populations, ensuring that treatments are both evidence-based and tailored to individual needs across a variety of clinical contexts.

Buoyancy, as described by Archimedes' principle, exerts an upward force on a submerged body, effectively reducing its weight. Since the human body's density (approximately $950kg/m^3$, or a specific gravity of approximately 0.974) is slightly lower than that of water, most individuals experience natural flotation, especially in denser water such as saltwater. This buoyant force significantly alters the biomechanical demands placed on the body, enabling therapeutic movements that may otherwise be difficult or impossible on land. The degree of weight off-loading depends on the depth of immersion: at pelvic depth, body weight is reduced by approximately 40%, at chest depth by about 60%, and at shoulder depth by up to 85% (Torres-Ronda & i del Alcázar, 2014). The level of buoyant support varies with immersion depth, allowing therapists to tailor exercises to individual needs. By carefully modulating immersion levels, clinicians can progressively challenge balance, strength, and coordination while maintaining safety and comfort. As a foundational component of rehabilitation, buoyancy provides a safer environment for individuals with mobility-related disabilities by reducing the risk of falls (Patil et al., 2024; Peng et al., 2025). It is particularly beneficial for those with arthritis, orthopaedic conditions, or neurological disabilities, as it minimises joint stress and enhances ease of movement (Mooventhan & Nivethitha, 2014).

Hydrostatic pressure, as described by Pascal's Law, increases proportionally with water depth and enhances circulation by promoting venous return and reducing oedema (Torres-Ronda & i del Alcázar, 2014). This uniform pressure acts consistently across the body's surface, providing an external stabilising force that assists in maintaining postural alignment during therapeutic activities. Immersion up to the neck increases central blood volume by approximately 30–35%, leading to elevated stroke volume and cardiac output, thereby supporting cardiovascular function and improving tissue perfusion (Torres-Ronda & i del Alcázar, 2014; Patil et al., 2024; Peng et al., 2025). This external compression also provides joint stabilisation and enhances proprioception by uniformly applying pressure to the body, reducing excessive movement while improving sensory feedback and postural control (Patil et al., 2024; Peng et al., 2025). These effects are particularly valuable for individuals with neurological conditions or musculoskeletal injuries, as they promote joint alignment and reduce discomfort during movement. Additionally, hydrostatic pressure can help alleviate pain, making therapeutic exercises more comfortable and effective (Patil et al., 2024; Peng et al., 2025). From a respiratory perspective, hydrostatic compression elevates the diaphragm and increases the resistance of inhalation. While this may require monitoring in individuals with respiratory conditions, it can also facilitate respiratory muscle training through controlled aquatic exercise (Torres-Ronda & i del Alcázar, 2014). Aquatic environments, therefore, provide unique opportunities for integrating cardiovascular, musculoskeletal, sensory, and respiratory rehabilitation into a single therapeutic session. These combined effects position hydrostatic pressure as a vital therapeutic element in circulatory, musculoskeletal, and respiratory rehabilitation.

Water's viscosity plays a fundamental role in hydrotherapy, offering consistent, multidirectional resistance that enhances muscle engagement and motor control (Torres-Ronda & i del Alcázar, 2014). This property distinguishes aquatic therapy environments from land-based settings, creating a dynamic medium in which every movement is met with supportive yet challenging resistance. Unlike on land, where resistance primarily opposes gravity, movement in water encounters resistance from all directions, making it an effective medium for strengthening, endurance training, and coordination while minimising impact-related strain (Patil et al., 2024; Peng et al., 2025). By enveloping the body uniformly, viscosity facilitates controlled and graded exercise opportunities suitable for a wide range of functional abilities.

The degree of resistance in water is influenced by movement speed, surface area, and turbulence. These factors interact to create a fluid, adjustable therapeutic environment, where slight changes in technique can significantly alter the exercise demands. At slower speeds or with streamlined motion, fluid flow remains laminar, while faster or broader movements produce turbulent flow and eddies, resulting in greater resistance. This shift from laminar to turbulent flow explains why small increases in velocity can exponentially increase the difficulty of aquatic movements. This fluid dynamic explains why viscosity increases resistance exponentially with velocity and how surface area shapes the total drag encountered. There are three primary types of drag forces in hydrotherapy: form drag, which occurs when water pressure differences create resistance in front of and behind a moving body; wave drag, generated by surface disturbances; and frictional drag, resulting from direct contact between the skin and water molecules (Torres-Ronda & i del Alcázar, 2014). By understanding these distinct forms of drag, clinicians can strategically design interventions that harness different resistance profiles to match therapeutic goals. These properties allow for precise modulation of exercise intensity by adjusting movement speed, body positioning, or incorporating aquatic equipment such as paddles or fins to increase resistance.

Notably, water's viscosity allows for immediate reduction in resistance when movement ceases, enabling individuals to self-regulate within their comfort zone. This instantaneous decrease in load provides an intuitive mechanism for adjusting effort without the need for external assistance, fostering autonomy and safety during therapy. This responsiveness supports what some researchers describe as an 'envelope of tolerance', a key benefit when working with individuals experiencing pain or neuromuscular limitations (Becker, 1994). Additionally, viscosity dampens momentum, slowing movement and providing individuals with more time to react and adjust their balance. This natural deceleration enhances postural control and provides critical support for practising complex motor tasks in a safer, more forgiving environment. This is particularly beneficial for those with coordination challenges, as it enhances proprioceptive feedback while supporting safe and controlled strengthening. Aquatic resistance training has been shown to improve muscle strength, aerobic capacity, flexibility, and functional movement across diverse populations (Torres-Ronda & i del Alcázar, 2014). As a result, the viscous resistance of water stands as a key therapeutic tool in hydrotherapy, underpinning interventions that are safe, adaptable, and capable of progressive advancement in accordance with individual rehabilitation needs.

The thermal properties of water play a crucial role in hydrotherapy, significantly enhancing its therapeutic benefits. Through its distinctive ability to regulate temperature and transfer heat efficiently, water provides a versatile and powerful medium for clinical interventions. Water's high specific heat capacity and thermal conductivity enable it to efficiently absorb and transfer heat, influencing both systemic and local physiological responses (Torres-Ronda & i del Alcázar, 2014). Unlike air, water facilitates more rapid heat exchange with the body, approximately 25 times faster, meaning immersion in warm or cold water can elicit widespread physiological effects beyond localised tissue changes (Espeland et al., 2022). This accelerated heat exchange allows hydrotherapy practitioners to achieve therapeutic goals more effectively, whether targeting circulatory, musculoskeletal, or sensory outcomes.

The optimal water temperature for therapeutic purposes varies depending on the intended outcome. Rehabilitation pools are generally maintained at 33.5–35.5°C, creating an environment that facilitates prolonged immersion without excessive thermal strain (Becker, 2009). Warmer aquatic settings, such as heated pools and hot tubs (37.5–41°C), support relaxation and muscle tension relief but may become uncomfortable over extended periods. Conversely, public and competitive swimming pools, typically kept at 27–29°C, are often too cool for rehabilitation participants engaging in lower-intensity movement. Such lower temperatures may limit muscular flexibility and could potentially exacerbate stiffness in individuals with musculoskeletal or neurological conditions. Cold water immersion, widely used in post-exercise recovery and inflammation management, generally ranges from 10–15°C (Becker, 2009; Espeland et al., 2022). Careful adjustment of water temperature thus becomes critical in matching therapeutic aims with the physiological responses elicited during immersion.

Warm-water immersion is particularly beneficial for individuals experiencing muscle stiffness, chronic pain, or circulatory challenges. It promotes vasodilation, enhances circulation, and reduces muscle tone, thereby alleviating discomfort and supporting mobility (Torres-Ronda & i del Alcázar, 2014). Since heat dissipates more rapidly in water than in air, immersion in warm water can increase skin temperature and lead to a slight rise in core body temperature, which in turn enhances blood flow and reduces muscle spasticity. This mechanism underpins many of the positive outcomes observed in hydrotherapy for individuals with conditions characterised by high muscle tone, such as cerebral palsy or post-stroke hemiparesis. Furthermore, warm water has a calming effect on sensory nerve endings, contributing to pain modulation and overall relaxation. In clinical hydrotherapy practice, water is typically maintained at a moderate but effective temperature of around 33°C, balancing the benefits of relaxation with the ability to engage in structured therapeutic exercises. Maintaining this moderate temperature ensures that sessions can focus on achieving rehabilitation goals without causing thermal fatigue or cardiovascular strain. In contrast, cold water immersion induces vasoconstriction, reduces inflammation, and provides analgesic effects, making it particularly useful for acute injury management and post-exercise recovery (Torres-Ronda & i del Alcázar, 2014). Cold water immersion also activates autonomic responses such as the cold shock response, characterised by an acute rise in heart rate, respiratory rate, and blood pressure, and the diving reflex, which includes a bradycardic response and peripheral vasoconstriction (Mooventhan & Nivethitha, 2014; Espeland et al., 2022). These physiological responses highlight the need for careful clinical judgment when incorporating cold water protocols, particularly among individuals with underlying cardiovascular vulnerabilities.

Repeated exposure to cold water may also yield long-term benefits, including enhanced cardiovascular efficiency, improved insulin sensitivity, reduced systemic inflammation, and increased thermogenic capacity via brown adipose tissue activation (Espeland et al., 2022). Warm-water immersion at moderate temperatures is particularly suitable for individuals managing chronic conditions, as it supports circulation, reduces muscle stiffness, and facilitates safe movement (Torres-Ronda & i del Alcázar, 2014; Becker, 2009).

These potential advantages support the inclusion of cold-water protocols within a personalised and supervised hydrotherapy programme. The ability to integrate both thermal stimulation and mechanical support through water-based therapy exemplifies the multidimensional capacity of hydrotherapy to address complex rehabilitation needs. The ability to manipulate water temperature, whether for warmth or cooling, makes it a valuable therapeutic tool for diverse populations. Warm water fosters muscle relaxation, comfort, and circulation, while cold water is effective for reducing acute inflammation and stimulating physiological alertness. Selecting the appropriate temperature is essential for optimising therapeutic outcomes and ensuring safe and effective hydrotherapy interventions (Patil et al., 2024; Peng et al., 2025).

Hydrodynamics, the study of how water moves and interacts with the body, is a fundamental knowledge in hydrotherapy. A thorough understanding of hydrodynamics enables clinicians to design aquatic interventions that strategically utilise water's physical forces to achieve specific therapeutic goals. Water flow patterns, such as laminar flow (smooth, uniform movement) and turbulent flow (chaotic, irregular currents), significantly influence resistance, stability, and movement control (Torres-Ronda & i del Alcázar, 2014). Laminar flow minimises resistance and facilitates smoother movement, whereas turbulent flow introduces instability and increased muscular demand, creating a dynamic therapeutic environment. Through careful observation of water behaviour, therapists can anticipate how movement patterns will alter resistance levels and postural demands. As individuals move through still water, they naturally generate turbulence, which increases resistance and proprioceptive feedback. Therapists can intentionally manipulate water flow by walking in front of or behind a participant, thereby generating currents that challenge balance, postural control, and neuromuscular engagement. These practitioner-induced currents provide an accessible means of progressing rehabilitation activities without altering pool equipment or water depth. Some therapeutic pools incorporate underwater treadmills or resistance jets, allowing individuals to train against moving water and enhance strength, endurance, and circulatory function. The controlled use of mechanical devices within aquatic environments further expands the range of therapeutic possibilities, supporting personalised and graded intervention planning.

A key hydrodynamic concept in hydrotherapy is streamlining, positioning the body to minimise drag. Maintaining a horizontal, streamlined posture reduces resistance and improves movement efficiency, whereas less streamlined positions increase drag due to greater surface area exposure (Torres-Ronda & i del Alcázar, 2014). Practising efficient body alignment in water not only optimises exercise but also fosters greater awareness of body positioning and movement economy. This principle is often applied in swimming-based rehabilitation, where proper body alignment not only enhances efficiency but also reduces energy expenditure. Additionally, wave dynamics can be therapeutically harnessed: movements near the surface generate waves that disrupt equilibrium and require continuous postural adjustments, thereby improving core stability and proprioceptive function. By intentionally engaging with wave-induced instability, therapists can challenge dynamic balance in a controlled and supportive setting.

Another critical hydrodynamic principle is the metacentric effect, which refers to the relationship between the centre of gravity and the centre of buoyancy and how it influences rotational stability in water (Becker, 2009). As body posture changes during immersion, the centre of buoyancy shifts relative to the centre of gravity. This creates subtle torque forces that continuously challenge balance and orientation. These forces act as constant stimuli for neuromuscular adaptation, requiring the individual to engage stabilising musculature and refine motor responses. These shifting buoyant forces provide rich sensory input to the nervous system, facilitating motor learning and adaptive responses. Therapists can leverage the metacentric effect to safely challenge postural control, enhancing neuromuscular coordination, proprioceptive awareness, and core activation across a range of functional levels. This natural interplay between gravitational and buoyant forces underpins many of the unique rehabilitation opportunities that aquatic environments offer.

A comprehensive understanding of these hydrodynamic principles allows therapists to tailor the level of challenge in hydrotherapy, ranging from gentle, still-water therapy for individuals with significant mobility needs to high-intensity, turbulent-water exercises for advanced rehabilitation. This ability to finely adjust the therapeutic environment according to individual capacity underscores hydrotherapy's flexibility and its applicability across a spectrum of presentations. This adaptability makes hydrotherapy a versatile and effective intervention for a diverse range of conditions and functional levels.

In summary, the properties of water, including buoyancy, hydrostatic pressure, viscosity (resistance), thermal effects, and hydrodynamics, form the scientific foundation of hydrotherapy. These fundamental principles interact dynamically to create an aquatic environment uniquely suited to rehabilitation and therapeutic exercise. They provide some advantages over land-based therapy, such as weight off-loading, natural resistance, 360-degree support and pressure, thermal modulation, and a safe environment for movement. By reducing gravitational loading, offering consistent multidirectional resistance, and facilitating controlled thermal and mechanical stimulation, water-based interventions address physical, sensory, and circulatory needs in ways that are difficult to replicate on land. The therapist's skill lies in harnessing these principles, for example by adjusting immersion depth, water temperature, or movement speed, to achieve specific therapeutic outcomes. Through careful and intentional manipulation of aquatic variables, clinicians can tailor hydrotherapy programmes to optimise functional recovery, enhance comfort, and promote long-term engagement in rehabilitation.

PHYSIOLOGICAL RESPONSES TO WATER IMMERSION

Immersion in water induces a cascade of physiological responses across multiple body systems, many of which contribute to its therapeutic benefits. These systemic effects, arising from the unique interaction between the human body and the aquatic environment, underpin much of the clinical value observed in hydrotherapy practice. These effects, particularly those associated with warm-water immersion and aquatic exercise, underpin the clinical advantages observed in individuals engaging in hydrotherapy. This section examines the impact of water immersion on the musculoskeletal, cardiovascular, nervous, respiratory, and immune systems, with a focus on how these physiological changes translate into improved functional outcomes. A multidimensional understanding of these mechanisms enables practitioners to maximise therapeutic benefits and promote holistic well-being through hydrotherapy.

Musculoskeletal System

Hydrotherapy provides substantial therapeutic benefits for the musculoskeletal system, primarily by reducing gravitational loading through buoyancy, thereby alleviating compressive stress on joints and the spine (Mooventhan & Nivethitha, 2014; Torres-Ronda & i del Alcázar, 2014). This unloading effect offers individuals the opportunity to experience movement with less discomfort and greater fluidity, particularly beneficial for those navigating musculoskeletal challenges. This unloading effect reduces pain and stiffness in weight-bearing joints, enhancing mobility and comfort for individuals with osteoarthritis, rheumatoid arthritis, and chronic low back pain.

Beyond buoyancy, hydrostatic pressure and water's thermal properties further contribute to musculoskeletal relief. The pressure exerted by water immersion aids in reducing post-injury and post-surgical edema, while the uniform warmth promotes muscle relaxation and enhances connective tissue extensibility (Mooventhan & Nivethitha, 2014). Together, these properties create an environment that supports joint flexibility, tissue healing, and functional ease. These combined effects support an increased range of motion (ROM) during aquatic exercise, often exceeding the flexibility gains achievable in land-based rehabilitation. A Cochrane systematic review on aquatic exercise for knee and hip osteoarthritis found statistically significant reductions in pain and disability, along with improvements in quality of life compared to non-exercise controls. Specifically, pain scores in hydrotherapy groups were, on average, five points lower on a 0–100 pain scale post-treatment, with measurable gains in functional mobility (Bartels et al., 2016). Similarly, for rheumatoid arthritis and chronic musculoskeletal pain conditions, water-based exercise appears to offer greater pain relief than conventional land-based therapy, particularly during ambulation. Many individuals with rheumatoid arthritis report experiencing greater ease and comfort in movement within the aquatic environment compared to land-based rehabilitation (Mooventhan & Nivethitha, 2014).

Beyond pain management, hydrotherapy serves as an effective intervention for muscle strengthening and endurance training, particularly for individuals for whom high-impact or weight-bearing exercises are contraindicated. Water's natural resistance allows for low-impact, progressive strengthening, enabling aquatic resistance exercises such as water walking, resistance training with flotation devices, and resistance paddles, all without placing undue stress on the joints. This makes hydrotherapy an accessible and sustainable exercise option for individuals across a wide range of physical abilities. Research indicates that aquatic training improves muscle power, endurance, and aerobic capacity, even among older adults and individuals undergoing rehabilitation (Torres-Ronda & i del Alcázar, 2014).

Hydrotherapy also supports early functional movement and gait training, as buoyancy reduces fall risk and provides partial weight support. This reduction in risk creates a safer environment for practising mobility skills, empowering individuals to regain confidence in their movements. This is particularly beneficial for individuals recovering from lower limb injuries or neurological conditions, such as stroke or spinal cord injury, where aquatic gait retraining enables mobility practice without requiring complex weight-support systems (Mooventhan & Nivethitha, 2014). Additionally, research suggests that buoyancy, combined with hydrostatic pressure, enhances proprioceptive input, potentially improving motor learning, ambulation confidence, and balance control (Torres-Ronda & i del Alcázar, 2014). Such enhancements contribute to more stable and efficient movement patterns, both within and beyond the aquatic setting.

Hydrotherapy has also been explored for spasticity management and muscle tone modulation, particularly in conditions such as stroke, cerebral palsy, and multiple sclerosis. Warm-water immersion is associated with reductions in spastic muscle tone, likely due to buoyancy-induced gravity reduction, thermal relaxation, and sustained sensory input (Mooventhan & Nivethitha, 2014). By softening the impact of spastic reflex activity, hydrotherapy facilitates smoother, more voluntary, and more coordinated movement experiences for individuals engaging in neurological rehabilitation. These factors may contribute to a reduction in spastic reflex activity, facilitating smoother and more voluntary movement patterns in neurological rehabilitation settings (Torres-Ronda & i del Alcázar, 2014).

In summary, hydrotherapy provides a multi-dimensional therapeutic approach for the musculoskeletal system, including pain reduction, decreased joint loading, enhanced joint mobility, muscle strengthening, and modulation of muscle tone. These physiological adaptations foster more effective functional movement, increased participation in daily activities, and enhanced overall rehabilitation outcomes across diverse populations.

Cardiovascular System

Hydrotherapy has significant effects on the cardiovascular system, primarily through hydrostatic pressure and reflex circulatory adjustments. These physiological responses, unique to immersion, form a central basis for the cardiovascular benefits observed in aquatic rehabilitation practices. When immersed to the chest or neck, hydrostatic pressure redistributes blood from the lower extremities and abdomen toward the thoracic cavity, increasing central blood volume by approximately 60%. This shift enhances venous return and increases cardiac stroke volume by approximately 35%, leading to a 30% rise in cardiac output with neck-level immersion, even in the absence of exercise (Becker, 2009). Such adaptations create an environment where circulatory efficiency is naturally optimised, even without active exertion.

At rest, heart rate may decrease slightly due to the diving reflex, particularly in cooler water, or remain stable. However, because stroke volume is elevated, overall cardiac output remains high. During aquatic exercise, maximum heart rate is typically lower than in land-based exercise at the same perceived effort, attributed to the combined effects of increased stroke volume and the cooling properties of water. This phenomenon enables individuals to engage in prolonged physical activity with reduced cardiovascular strain, supporting exercise participation even among those with limited land-based endurance. This results in a more efficient cardiovascular response, allowing individuals with cardiovascular limitations to exercise for longer durations with lower perceived exertion (Torres-Ronda & i del Alcázar, 2014).

Water temperature plays a crucial role in cardiovascular function. Warm water immersion induces peripheral vasodilation, increasing cutaneous blood flow and cardiac output as the body dissipates heat. Conversely, cold water immersion initially triggers a rise in blood pressure and heart rate due to sympathetic activation, followed by a reflex bradycardic response with prolonged exposure (Mooventhan & Nivethitha, 2014). Understanding these thermal effects is essential for safely designing aquatic interventions, particularly for individuals managing cardiovascular health conditions. These temperature-related effects are particularly relevant for individuals with hypertension, heart failure, or circulatory disorders, necessitating careful monitoring of immersion parameters.

Hydrotherapy has been explored as a complementary intervention in cardiac rehabilitation. Research suggests that aquatic aerobic exercise, such as deep-water running or water jogging, can improve VO_2max and cardiovascular endurance in individuals with low to moderate fitness levels similarly to land-based training (Torres-Ronda & i del Alcázar, 2014). The aquatic environment, through its combined effects of buoyancy and thermal regulation, provides an accessible platform for safe and sustainable cardiovascular conditioning. The buoyancy and cooling effects of water enable individuals with limited cardiovascular tolerance on land to sustain exercise for longer periods at a reduced heart rate.

For individuals with chronic heart failure, hydrotherapy has shown potential benefits, including enhanced circulatory function, improved exercise tolerance, and reduced sympathetic tone following warm-water exercise (Mooventhan & Nivethitha, 2014). However, caution is required for individuals with severe heart failure or unstable cardiovascular conditions, as the autotransfusion effect of immersion significantly increases cardiac preload and central volume load. When appropriately monitored in a clinical setting, this physiological response may be harnessed to support haemodynamic function and functional recovery. When administered in a controlled clinical setting, this volume shift may actually be beneficial, and some cardiac rehabilitation programmes incorporate hydrotherapy to optimise haemodynamic function while minimising weight-bearing strain (Mooventhan & Nivethitha, 2014).

Additionally, hydrostatic pressure aids peripheral circulation by reducing venous stasis and oedema, benefiting individuals with chronic venous insufficiency or limb swelling (Torres-Ronda & i del Alcázar, 2014). The compression exerted by water stimulates a mild diuretic effect (increased urine output) due to central volume expansion and the release of atrial natriuretic peptide, which may assist in fluid regulation and blood pressure control (Becker, 2009). Such effects further highlight hydrotherapy's multifaceted role in promoting cardiovascular and circulatory health across a range of clinical presentations.

In summary, hydrotherapy offers multiple cardiovascular benefits, including enhanced cardiac output, reduced heart rate response for a given workload, improved circulation, and decreased systemic vascular resistance. These physiological adaptations collectively support hydrotherapy's value as a safe, effective, and adaptable intervention in cardiac rehabilitation, hypertension management, and vascular health promotion for diverse populations.

Nervous System

Hydrotherapy exerts multifaceted effects on the nervous system, influencing both central and peripheral mechanisms through sensory stimulation, autonomic modulation, and neuroplasticity-related adaptations. These complex interactions contribute to hydrotherapy's unique ability to support neurological rehabilitation and psychological well-being.

One of the primary mechanisms by which hydrotherapy impacts the nervous system is through sensory nerve activation. Mechanoreceptors in the skin are continuously stimulated by hydrostatic pressure and the dynamic movement of water across the body, leading to enhanced sensory feedback (Becker, 2020). The warmth of therapeutic pools further activates thermoreceptors, promoting comfort and relaxation. Together, these sensory inputs foster a supportive environment for modulating pain perception, enhancing proprioception, and facilitating relaxation. These combined effects explain why individuals undergoing warm-water therapy frequently report reductions in pain, muscle spasms, and soreness, which are likely mediated by thermal and pressure-related suppression of nociceptive input and reduced muscle spindle excitability (Mooventhan & Nivethitha, 2014).

Hydrotherapy also induces significant changes in autonomic nervous system activity, primarily by shifting autonomic balance toward parasympathetic dominance, the 'rest and digest' response. Studies on heart rate variability indicate that warm water immersion increases vagal tone, reflecting a relaxation response (Rodica-Georgeta & Gheorghe, 2022). Certain aquatic therapy techniques, such as Watsu, have been developed explicitly to suppress sympathetic activity and enhance parasympathetic regulation (Rodica-Georgeta & Gheorghe, 2022). These autonomic shifts are often accompanied by reductions in cortisol levels and improvements in psychological well-being, highlighting hydrotherapy's integrative role in physical and emotional health. These autonomic adjustments are supported by reduced cortisol levels and improved mood states, making hydrotherapy particularly beneficial for individuals experiencing stress-related muscle tension or psychosomatic pain. In contrast, cold water immersion transiently activates the sympathetic nervous system, causing a surge in noradrenaline, increased alertness, and an acute rise in blood pressure and heart rate. Over time, repeated cold exposure may enhance sympathetic stability and stress resilience, a process associated with hormesis, though its application in clinical hydrotherapy is primarily limited to athletic recovery and specific therapeutic conditions (Mooventhan & Nivethitha, 2014).

Hydrotherapy also affects cerebral circulation, as immersion up to the clavicle has been shown to enhance cerebral blood flow due to increased cardiac output and improved carotid artery perfusion (Becker, 2020). Increased brain perfusion during aquatic exercise may contribute to cognitive benefits and emotional regulation, particularly valuable for individuals managing neurological or neurodegenerative conditions. This increase in brain perfusion may underlie some of the cognitive and neurological benefits of aquatic exercise, particularly in populations with neurodegenerative disorders such as Parkinson's disease, where autonomic dysregulation and stress-related symptoms can be alleviated through aquatic therapy (Becker, 2020). Furthermore, water-based exercise has been linked to neuronal plasticity and cognitive improvements, suggesting potential applications in neurorehabilitation and cognitive therapy (Nissim et al., 2018, 2021).

In the context of neurological rehabilitation, hydrotherapy provides a controlled yet enriched sensory-motor environment that can benefit individuals with neurological conditions such as stroke, traumatic brain injury, or cerebral palsy. The aquatic environment facilitates graduated movement challenges, enabling the safe exploration of postural adjustments and dynamic balance strategies without the fear of falling. The buoyancy of water reduces gravitational constraints, allowing for controlled postural adjustments and balance training without fall risk. The Halliwick method, for example, employs controlled instability and water-based righting reactions to facilitate motor relearning and neuromuscular adaptation (Rodica-Georgeta & Gheorghe, 2022). A systematic review on stroke rehabilitation found that incorporating aquatic therapy improved walking ability, balance, emotional well-being, and overall quality of life compared to land-based therapy alone (Veldema & Jansen, 2021). Additionally, warm water immersion has been shown to reduce muscle spasticity, likely due to reduced spinal reflex excitability and muscle hypertonicity (Veldema & Jansen, 2021).

Beyond direct neurological effects, hydrotherapy offers psychological benefits that intersect with neurophysiological mechanisms. The combination of buoyancy, warmth, and hydrostatic pressure creates a sensory-rich, low-gravity environment that reduces anxiety and enhances well-being. Individuals engaging in aquatic therapy often report improvements in mood, self-confidence, and emotional resilience, reinforcing the holistic benefits of water-based interventions. Individuals with chronic pain, neurological conditions, or anxiety-related conditions frequently exhibit improvements in mood and self-confidence following group-based or one-on-one aquatic therapy. These emotional benefits may be partially attributed to exercise-induced endorphin release, increased parasympathetic activity, and modulation of neurotransmitter levels (Mooventhan & Nivethitha, 2014).

Hydrotherapy exerts broad and clinically significant effects on the nervous system, including pain modulation, autonomic regulation, improved sensory-motor function, and enhanced cerebral perfusion. These effects reflect hydrotherapy's capacity to address multiple dimensions of well-being simultaneously, encompassing physical, cognitive, and emotional domains. These physiological mechanisms underpin its benefits for individuals with chronic pain, fibromyalgia, stroke, spinal cord injury, multiple sclerosis, Parkinson's disease, and other neuromuscular conditions. As ongoing research explores the relationship between hydrotherapy, neuroplasticity, and cognitive function, hydrotherapy continues to emerge as a valuable modality in neurological and psychological rehabilitation.

In summary, hydrotherapy may influence the nervous system through a combination of sensory stimulation, autonomic regulation, pain modulation, and cognitive enhancement. By providing consistent tactile input, promoting parasympathetic activation, and creating an inclusive and supportive environment for motor relearning, hydrotherapy offers a unique and person-centred therapeutic opportunity for individuals across a range of neurological and psychological profiles.

Respiratory System

Hydrotherapy exerts significant effects on the respiratory system, primarily due to hydrostatic pressure and immersion depth. These effects arise from the unique interaction between external water pressure and thoracic mechanics, influencing respiratory effort and ventilatory capacity. When an individual is immersed in chest- or neck-deep water, the external pressure exerted on the thorax and abdomen increases, restricting lung expansion and elevating the work of breathing (Torres-Ronda & i del Alcázar, 2014). As a result, vital capacity decreases, as the lungs must work against external hydrostatic pressure to expand. Becker (2009) reports that immersion to shoulder or neck depth significantly reduces vital capacity, with warm water further amplifying this effect due to increased peripheral vasodilation and thoracic blood volume.

Despite the increased resistance, tidal volume (the air exchanged per breath) may initially increase as a compensatory mechanism, particularly during cool water immersion. This adaptive response helps maintain gas exchange and ventilatory efficiency during immersion, although it is limited by lung compliance and individual tolerance. Overall, water immersion elevates the work of breathing by approximately 60% compared to standing on land, primarily because the diaphragm and intercostal muscles must overcome external hydrostatic resistance (Becker, 2009). While this added effort may pose challenges for individuals with severe respiratory conditions such as advanced chronic obstructive pulmonary disease (COPD) or restrictive lung disease, it may also serve as a training stimulus for respiratory muscles, improving breathing efficiency over time (Torres-Ronda & i del Alcázar, 2014). Such training effects may contribute to improved functional capacity and endurance when appropriately dosed and supervised.

Beyond its mechanical effects, hydrotherapy has been associated with respiratory benefits, particularly in the context of mucus mobilisation and airway hydration.

Warm water immersion, combined with physical activity, may aid in airway clearance for individuals with certain respiratory conditions by promoting secretion mobilisation and enhancing mucociliary function. These outcomes may support more effective pulmonary hygiene and comfort during therapy sessions. Additionally, immersion in a warm, humid environment may help maintain airway hydration, although its effects can vary among individuals. While some individuals with chronic respiratory conditions benefit from humid environments, others, particularly those with asthma, may experience symptom exacerbation due to airway reactivity (Mooventhan & Nivethitha, 2014). This variability highlights the importance of personalising aquatic interventions based on individual respiratory profiles.

Cold water immersion elicits two concurrent but distinct physiological responses: the cold shock response and the diving response. The cold shock response, triggered primarily by rapid skin cooling, involves an immediate inspiratory gasp, tachycardia, hyperventilation, and sympathetic activation, significantly increasing cardiac workload and ventilatory drive. In contrast, the diving response, typically triggered by facial immersion, induces bradycardia, apnoea, and selective peripheral vasoconstriction, aiming to preserve oxygen for vital organs (Tipton, 1989). While these reflexes are protective in certain contexts, they may also pose risks, particularly for individuals with pre-existing cardiovascular or respiratory vulnerabilities. These opposing autonomic responses underscore the complex physiological interactions between cold water immersion and respiratory function.

For most individuals, moderate immersion (waist or chest level) does not significantly impair breathing function and may even contribute to respiratory muscle training by increasing the work of breathing. However, careful adjustments to immersion depth and activity intensity are necessary for individuals with respiratory limitations to ensure safety and optimal benefits (Mooventhan & Nivethitha, 2014). Individualised monitoring and pacing strategies are critical to maximising therapeutic outcomes while avoiding respiratory fatigue.

Notably, repeated cold water exposure has been linked to immunological adaptations, such as enhanced leukocyte activity and increased natural killer (NK) cell function, particularly when preceded by moderate exercise. These immune changes may contribute to improved respiratory health and reduced susceptibility to infections in certain populations, supporting the notion that controlled cold water immersion could serve as an adjunctive approach in respiratory rehabilitation (Brenner et al., 1999). This emerging evidence highlights the potential for integrating hydrotherapy into broader strategies for supporting respiratory and immune function.

Hydrotherapy presents both challenges and benefits for respiratory function. While hydrostatic pressure increases mechanical resistance, this effect can serve as a training stimulus for respiratory muscles, strengthening the diaphragm and intercostals. When delivered within appropriate clinical parameters, this form of resistance may support improvements in ventilatory strength and efficiency. With appropriate clinical modifications and careful monitoring, hydrotherapy can be a safe and effective intervention for many individuals with respiratory conditions. However, contraindications such as uncontrolled asthma or severely restricted vital capacity must be carefully considered to ensure safety. A person-centred approach, based on individual tolerance and needs, is essential to guiding safe aquatic respiratory rehabilitation.

Immune and Endocrine System

Hydrotherapy's influence on immune function and endocrine regulation has gained increasing attention (Mooventhan & Nivethitha, 2014). The complex interaction between thermal stimulation, nervous system activation, and hormonal modulation provides a basis for understanding these systemic effects. Research suggests that regular water immersion, particularly cold water exposure, may act as a mild physiological stressor, stimulating immune responses and adaptive resilience (Brenner et al., 1999; Shevchuk, 2007).

Cold water immersion has been associated with acute increases in white blood cell counts, particularly neutrophils and lymphocytes, alongside enhanced natural killer (NK) cell activity (Brenner et al., 1999). Experimental studies indicate that repeated brief cold water exposure leads to elevated cytokine levels, including interleukin-6 (IL-6) and gamma-interferon, suggesting a transient enhancement of immune function (Shevchuk, 2007). Additionally, in individuals with COPD, repeated cold water exposure has been linked to a reduced frequency of respiratory infections and improved immune markers, possibly due to immune surveillance enhancement and inflammatory modulation (Goedsche et al., 2007). These findings support the therapeutic interest in cold water protocols for selected populations, particularly where immune robustness is a clinical priority.

The underlying mechanisms for these cold-induced immune responses involve sympathetic nervous system activation and the hypothalamic-pituitary-adrenal (HPA) axis, leading to the release of catecholamines and glucocorticoids, which in turn mobilise immune cells into circulation (Brenner et al., 1999). Some researchers propose that repeated cold exposure may function as a form of 'immune training', enhancing immune vigilance over time. Furthermore, there is speculation that cold-induced immune stimulation may play a role in anti-tumour immunity, although this remains largely theoretical and requires further investigation

(Shevchuk, 2007). While preliminary data are promising, additional studies are needed to clarify the clinical relevance of these responses.

In contrast, warm-water immersion exerts a distinct modulatory effect on the endocrine stress response. Immersion in thermoneutral or warm water is associated with reduced cortisol levels, increased endorphin release, and improved autonomic balance, which may contribute to pain relief, enhanced mood, and relaxation (Mooventhan & Nivethitha, 2014; Shevchuk, 2008). These effects support the use of warm-water hydrotherapy in contexts where stress reduction and emotional regulation are therapeutic goals. By attenuating chronic stress and improving sleep quality, both factors known to influence immune suppression, warm hydrotherapy may indirectly support immune function (Blazickova et al., 2000). This indirect immune benefit reinforces the integrative value of hydrotherapy in long-term health management.

Additionally, aquatic exercise has been linked to enhanced blood and lymphatic circulation, potentially facilitating immune cell trafficking and optimising immune surveillance throughout the body (Mooventhan & Nivethitha, 2014). Some balneotherapy studies (therapeutic mineral baths) have reported reductions in inflammatory markers in individuals with rheumatoid arthritis following a course of thermal mineral water therapy, suggesting potential anti-inflammatory effects (Yurtkuran et al., 2006). While further research is needed, these findings support hydrotherapy's potential to modulate systemic inflammation in chronic conditions.

Hydrotherapy exerts systemic effects on immune and endocrine function, with cold water immersion stimulating acute immune responses, potentially leading to fewer infections and heightened immune activity in specific contexts. Meanwhile, warm-water therapies promote stress reduction and anti-inflammatory effects, indirectly benefiting immune regulation and homeostasis. Together, these multi-systemic effects highlight the therapeutic versatility of hydrotherapy and its ability to address interconnected physical and psychological domains. These multisystemic benefits, combined with hydrotherapy's therapeutic effects on other physiological systems, highlight its holistic rehabilitative potential.

The next section will explore the practical applications of hydrotherapy, detailing general aquatic exercise approaches as well as specialised methodologies such as Watsu and the Halliwick concept, which have been designed to address specific rehabilitation objectives. These structured interventions demonstrate how the physiological principles outlined throughout this section are translated into targeted, evidence-based strategies that meet the diverse needs of individuals in rehabilitation settings.

TECHNIQUES IN HYDROTHERAPY

Hydrotherapy encompasses a diverse range of approaches that utilise the unique properties of water to support health, rehabilitation, and overall well-being. These approaches address a variety of needs, including pain management, mobility support, neuromuscular coordination, and cardiovascular conditioning. The selection of a hydrotherapy method depends on the individual's goals, preferences, and therapeutic needs, as well as on available resources such as therapy pools, specialised equipment, and trained aquatic therapists.

Broadly, hydrotherapy techniques can be categorised into active and passive (or therapist-facilitated) approaches, each offering distinct benefits. This classification helps guide clinical decision-making and facilitates appropriate matching between method and participant.

Active hydrotherapy includes approaches in which individuals actively participate in guided movement within the water. The buoyancy, resistance, and support provided by water allow for safe and accessible movement, making aquatic exercise particularly beneficial for people with diverse mobility levels. Structured programmes, such as deep water running and Ai Chi (a water-based adaptation of Tai Chi), help individuals enhance strength, flexibility, coordination, and endurance in a way that reduces impact on joints and muscles (Lambeck & Bommer, 2010; Oddsson, 2019). These activities combine therapeutic benefit with functional training, creating opportunities for gradual progression within a supportive setting. These activities can be tailored to accommodate different abilities and support a range of rehabilitation and fitness goals.

Passive hydrotherapy techniques focus on providing support, relaxation, and facilitated movement without requiring active participation. These approaches can be particularly helpful for individuals who experience pain, muscle stiffness, or limited ability to initiate movement independently. Examples include Watsu, which combines elements of Shiatsu massage and assisted floating, and AquaStretch, which uses gentle guided movement to promote joint mobility and reduce muscular tension (Schitter et al., 2020; Patil et al., 2024). These methods emphasise presence, responsiveness, and sensory connection, contributing to a calming therapeutic experience.

Both active and passive hydrotherapy methods offer unique advantages, and in many cases, they are combined to create a comprehensive and person-centred approach to hydrotherapy. While active methods can promote strength-building, endurance, and motor coordination, passive techniques provide valuable opportunities for pain relief, stress reduction, and movement facilitation in a supported environment. The integration of both approaches enables therapists to tailor interventions that align with physical capacity, emotional state, and therapeutic goals.

The following sections will explore several hydrotherapy methods, outlining their practical applications, core techniques, and the research supporting their effectiveness in diverse therapeutic contexts. By linking theory with practice, these examples will demonstrate how water-based methods can be applied in inclusive and evidence-informed ways across a range of populations and needs.

The Halliwick Concept

Originally developed by James McMillan in the 1940s to support individuals with disabilities in learning to swim, the Halliwick Concept has since evolved into a structured aquatic therapy approach emphasising motor control, postural stability, and balance retraining. Grounded in inclusive principles, the approach is designed to empower participants through progressive mastery of movement within the aquatic environment. At its core is the Ten-Point Programme, which systematically guides participants through water adaptation, rotational control, and movement coordination, ultimately fostering greater independence in aquatic environments (Lambeck & Gamper, 2011). The Ten-Point Programme provides a logical framework that supports gradual skill acquisition, building confidence and functional competence at each stage.

This approach is widely utilised in neurological and paediatric rehabilitation, particularly for individuals with cerebral palsy, autism spectrum disorder, and other conditions affecting balance and sensory-motor integration. By addressing foundational movement skills in a supportive, low-gravity environment, the Halliwick Concept facilitates both physical development and psychological engagement. By leveraging the unique properties of water, the Halliwick Concept promotes body awareness, controlled movement, and functional mobility, making it a valuable tool for a broad range of therapeutic applications. Its adaptability across ages and functional levels further underscores its significance within contemporary aquatic therapy practice.

The Bad Ragaz Ring Method (BRRM)

Originally developed in Switzerland in the 1960s, the Bad Ragaz Ring Method (BRRM) applies proprioceptive neuromuscular facilitation (PNF) principles within an aquatic environment. Drawing on established land-based rehabilitation strategies,

BRRM adapts these techniques to leverage the supportive and resistive properties of water. Individuals are supported by flotation rings while a therapist provides graded resistance and guided movement patterns to facilitate neuromuscular activation and control. The use of buoyancy aids enables participants to maintain a horizontal position, freeing the therapist to focus on movement quality and targeted facilitation.

This approach is particularly beneficial for improving muscular strength, postural stability, and neuromuscular coordination, making it a valuable intervention in musculoskeletal and neurological rehabilitation (Gamper & Lambeck, 2011; Patil et al., 2024). Its structured yet adaptable format allows therapists to modulate exercise intensity, providing both gentle activation for early-stage recovery and more challenging resistance training for advanced rehabilitation goals. Through precise therapist-guided interventions, BRRM supports functional gains while minimising the impact forces associated with land-based therapy.

Ai Chi

Developed by Jun Konno in 1993, Ai Chi is a water-based movement therapy that integrates principles from Tai Chi and Qi Gong with breath synchronisation in shoulder-depth warm water. Drawing inspiration from ancient movement traditions, Ai Chi adapts these principles to the aquatic environment, creating a fluid practice. This method consists of 19 slow, controlled, and continuous movements, gradually transitioning from upper-body to full-body engagement, with an emphasis on balance, energy flow, and postural control (Lambeck & Bommer, 2010). The mindful coordination of breathing and movement forms the foundation of Ai Chi's therapeutic potential, promoting an integrated physical and mental focus throughout the practice.

Ai Chi promotes relaxation, enhances neuromuscular coordination, and improves flexibility while fostering a mindful connection between movement and breath. The soothing properties of warm water further enhance the sensory experience, facilitating emotional calmness alongside physical rehabilitation.

Therapeutically, Ai Chi has been shown to benefit people with neurological conditions, chronic pain, respiratory challenges, and balance difficulties. Research suggests that the combination of buoyancy, resistance, and deep breathing contributes to reduced stress levels, improved respiratory efficiency, and enhanced postural stability, making it a valuable approach for supporting balance and mobility (Lambeck & Bommer, 2010; Nissim et al., 2021; Patil et al., 2024). Its structured yet adaptable format allows individuals to engage with therapeutic movement at their own pace, aligning physical rehabilitation with psychological well-being.

Deep Water Running (DWR)

Deep Water Running (DWR) is an aquatic training technique that replicates land-based running patterns while the participant is suspended in deep water using flotation belts or vests. By eliminating ground impact, DWR allows individuals to engage in dynamic aerobic exercise within a supportive, low-gravity environment. This method facilitates cardiovascular conditioning and lower limb muscle activation without placing stress on weight-bearing joints. The resistance provided by the surrounding water offers continuous muscular engagement, enhancing both endurance and neuromuscular control.

DWR is widely used in rehabilitation programmes for individuals recovering from lower-limb injuries, as well as in athletic training and general fitness. Its versatility makes it an appealing option across rehabilitation, performance maintenance, and cross-training contexts. It offers a safe and effective alternative for maintaining endurance, neuromuscular coordination, and functional mobility during recovery (Patil et al., 2024). Furthermore, by enabling high-intensity cardiovascular exercise with minimal joint loading, DWR supports both physical conditioning and injury prevention strategies.

Rehabilitation Swimming

Rehabilitation Swimming utilises swimming as a therapeutic intervention, providing a low-impact, full-body exercise that supports cardiovascular fitness, muscular strength, and mobility. By harnessing the inherent buoyancy and resistance of water, this approach facilitates dynamic movement while minimising the stresses typically associated with weight-bearing exercise. This method is particularly beneficial for individuals seeking a safe and adaptive approach to movement, as it minimises joint stress while promoting functional recovery. It enables participants to engage in meaningful physical activity while protecting vulnerable structures, such as joints, tendons, and the spine.

Rehabilitation swimming has also been recognised as an effective transition to adaptive sports and competitive swimming programmes for individuals with disabilities, fostering physical confidence and participation in aquatic activities (Moffatt, 2017; Aitchison et al., 2020).

An emerging approach within rehabilitation swimming is the Water World Swimming Therapy method, developed by Ori Sela, which focuses on modifying swimming techniques to reduce strain on the neck and lower back. This method integrates hydrotherapy principles with traditional swimming practices, creating a more individualised and responsive aquatic experience. It emphasises fluid, gentle movements that align with an individual's physical needs, thereby supporting both therapeutic goals and personal comfort. By adapting swimming styles to accommodate specific functional ability, Water World Swimming Therapy broadens access to aquatic rehabilitation and promotes long-term engagement in water-based physical activity.

Watsu

Developed by Harold Dull in the 1980s, Watsu is a passive hydrotherapy that combines principles of Shiatsu massage, myofascial stretching, and joint mobilisation in a thermoneutral water environment (approximately 35°C). By merging manual therapy techniques with the supportive properties of water, Watsu offers a unique integrative therapeutic experience. The therapist supports the participant in a supine floating position, facilitating gentle, rhythmic movements that promote deep relaxation, reduce muscular tension, and enhance joint mobility. The continuous sensory feedback provided by the water environment contributes to a profound sense of comfort and safety, enabling deeper physical and emotional release.

The unique sensory experience of Watsu has been found to contribute to both physical and psychological well-being. Systematic reviews and meta-analyses indicate that Watsu is associated with significant reductions in pain, improvements in physical function, and positive effects on mental health and sleep quality. These outcomes suggest that Watsu can effectively address multidimensional aspects of well-being, bridging physical rehabilitation with emotional support. Research has demonstrated its benefits for individuals with musculoskeletal conditions, neurological impairments such as cerebral palsy and stroke, and chronic pain syndromes, as well as in supportive care settings, including palliative care (Schitter et al., 2020).

AquaStretch

AquaStretch is an aquatic therapy technique that integrates elements of assisted stretching, myofascial release, and active movement in a gravity-reduced water environment. Conducted in shallow water with weighted resistance, AquaStretch is a highly interactive method, as participants are encouraged to communicate sensations of tension and release with the therapist to guide the treatment process effectively.

AquaStretch reduces joint compression and allows individuals to achieve movement patterns that may be difficult to perform in a weight-bearing environment. The aquatic setting facilitates safe exploration of mobility without exacerbating mechanical strain. The immersion in warm water plays a critical role in the technique's efficacy, increasing blood flow to muscles by over 50% and enhancing tissue elasticity, which can facilitate deeper stretching with minimal discomfort. This physiological environment supports gentle yet effective neuromuscular adaptation, optimising outcomes for flexibility and joint function.

This combination of warmth, hydrostatic pressure, and reduced gravitational forces enables participants to experience improved flexibility, reduced musculoskeletal restriction, and increased joint range of motion (Sherlock et al., 2013). Emerging clinical applications of AquaStretch suggest its potential benefits for individuals experiencing chronic pain, movement restrictions, and postural imbalances. Early studies indicate that even a single session may yield measurable improvements in mobility and movement efficiency (Culea & Simion, 2022).

Hydrotherapy techniques range from active aquatic exercise to passive relaxation-based interventions, with specialised approaches tailored for neurological, musculoskeletal, and cardiovascular rehabilitation. Aquatic exercise programmes offer a structured means of improving strength, endurance, and mobility, promoting functional gains across diverse populations. While passive therapies such as Watsu focus on relaxation and pain relief, methods like the Halliwick Concept provide structured motor learning strategies that foster postural control and independence.

As research continues to explore hydrotherapy's clinical applications, new evidence-based techniques are emerging, further expanding its role in modern rehabilitation practice. By combining scientific principles with the unique properties of water, hydrotherapy offers a holistic platform for physical, neurological, and emotional restoration.

REFERENCES

Aitchison, B., Soundy, A., Martin, P., Rushton, A., & Heneghan, N. R. (2020). Lived experiences of social support in Paralympic swimmers: A protocol for a qualitative study. *BMJ Open*, *10*(9), e039953.

Bartels, E. M., Juhl, C. B., Christensen, R., Hagen, K. B., Danneskiold-Samsøe, B., Dagfinrud, H., & Lund, H. (2016). Aquatic exercise for the treatment of knee and hip osteoarthritis. *Cochrane Database of Systematic Reviews*, *3*(3), 1–52.

Becker, B. E. (1994). The biologic aspects of hydrotherapy. *Journal of Back and Musculoskeletal Rehabilitation*, *4*(4), 255–264.

Becker, B. E. (2009). Aquatic therapy: Scientific foundations and clinical rehabilitation applications. *PM&R*, *1*(9), 859–872.

Becker, B. E. (2020). Aquatic therapy in contemporary neurorehabilitation: An update. *PM&R*, *12*(12), 1251–1259

Bender, T., Balint, P. V., & Balint, G. P. (2002). A brief history of spa therapy. *Annals of the Rheumatic Diseases*, *61*(10), 949–950.

Blazickova, S., Rovenský, J., Koska, J., & Vigas, M. (2000). Effect of hyperthermic water bath on parameters of cellular immunity. *International Journal of Clinical Pharmacology Research*, *20*(1–2), 41–46.

Brenner, I. K. M., Castellani, J. W., Gabaree, C., Young, A. J., Zamecnik, J., Shephard, R. J., & Shek, P. N. (1999). Immune changes in humans during cold exposure: Effects of prior heating and exercise. *Journal of Applied Physiology*, *87*, 699–710.

Brody, L. T., & Geigle, P. R. (eds). (2009). *Aquatic Exercise for Rehabilitation and Training*. Human Kinetics.

Burns, S. B., & Burns, J. L. (1997). Hydrotherapy. *The Journal of Alternative and Complementary Medicine*, *3*(2), 105–107.

Cole, A. J. & Becker, B. E. (2004). *Comprehensive Aquatic Therapy*. Butterworth Heinemann.

Culea, R. G., & Simion, G. (2022). Aquatic therapy: Some theoretical considerations about Bad Ragaz Ring Method. *Science, Movement and Health*, *22*(2), 119–126.

De Vierville, J. P. (1997). Aquatic rehabilitation: An historical perspective. In *Comprehensive Aquatic Therapy* (1st edn, pp. 1–16). Butterworth-Heinemann.

Espeland, D., de Weerd, L., & Mercer, J. B. (2022). Health effects of voluntary exposure to cold water–a continuing subject of debate. *International Journal of Circumpolar Health*, *81*(1), 2111789.

Fields, A. (1950). Physiotherapy in ancient Chinese medicine. *The American Journal of Surgery*, *79*(4), 613–616.

Gamper, U., & Lambeck, J. (2011). The Bad Ragaz Ring Method. In J. Lambeck & U. Gamper (eds), *Comprehensive Aquatic Therapy* (3rd edn, pp. 109–136). Washington State University Publishing.

Goedsche, K., Förster, M., Kroegel, C., & Uhlemann, C. (2007). Repeated cold water stimulations (hydrotherapy according to Kneipp) in patients with COPD. *Forschende Komplementarmedizin*, *14*(3), 158–166.

Irion, J. M. (1997). Historical overview of aquatic rehabilitation. *Aquatic Rehabilitation*, 3–13.

Lambeck, J., & Bommer, A. (2010). Ai Chi®: Applications in clinical practice. In *Comprehensive Aquatic Therapy* (3rd edn). Washington State University Publishing.

Lambeck, J., & Gamper, U. N. (2011). The Halliwick concept. In J. Lambeck & U. Gamper (eds), *Comprehensive Aquatic Therapy* (3rd edn). Washington State University Publishing.

Moffatt, F. (2017). The individual physical health benefits of swimming: a literature review. *The Health & Wellbeing Benefits of Swimming*, 8–25.

Mooventhan, A., & Nivethitha, L. (2014). Scientific evidence-based effects of hydrotherapy on various systems of the body. *North American Journal of Medical Sciences*, *6*(5), 199–209.

Nissim, M., Ram-Tsur, R., Glicksohn, J., Zion, M., Mevarech, Z., Harpaz, Y., & Dotan Ben-Soussan, T. (2018). Effects of aquatic motor intervention on verbal working memory and brain activity: A pilot study. *Mind, Brain and Education*, *12*(2), 71–81. https://doi.org/10.1111/mbe.12174

Nissim, M., Livny, A., Barmatz, C., Tsarfaty, G., Berner, Y., Sacher, Y., & Ratzon, N. Z. (2021). Effects of Ai-Chi practice on balance and left cerebellar activation during high working memory load task in older people: A controlled pilot trial. *International Journal of Environmental Research and Public Health, 18*(23), 12756.

Oddsson, E. E. (2019). Effects of deep-water running and land-based running program on aerobic power, physical fitness and motivation on female youth footballers (Doctoral dissertation).

Patil, C., Patil, P., & Fernandez, C. (2024). Aquatic therapy in contemporary neurorehabilitation. *African Journal of Biological Sciences, 6*(Si3), 1755–1760.

Peng, Y., Zou, Y., & Asakawa, T. (2025). The glamor of and insights regarding hydrotherapy, from simple immersion to advanced computer-assisted exercises: A narrative review. *BioScience Trends*, 2024–01356.

Ring, J. W. (1996). Windows, baths, and solar energy in the Roman empire. *American Journal of Archaeology, 100*(4), 717–724.

Rodica-Georgeta, C. & Gheorghe, S. (2022). Investigations regarding the opinions of the specialists on the knowledges of the Bad Ragaz Ring Method. *Ovidius University Annals, Series Physical Education & Sport/Science, Movement & Health, 22*(2), 127–133.

Schitter, A. M., Fleckenstein, J., Frei, P., Taeymans, J., Kurpiers, N., & Radlinger, L. (2020). Applications, indications, and effects of passive hydrotherapy WATSU (WaterShiatsu): A systematic review and meta-analysis. *PLoS One, 15*(3), e0229705.

Sherlock, L. A., & Eversaul, G. (2013). The effects of a single AquaStretch™ session on lower extremity range of motion. In *Poster presented at the International Aquatic Fitness Conference (2013, May), Orlando, FL and World Aquatic Health Conference (2013, Oct), Indianapolis, IN.*

Shevchuk, N. A. (2007). Possible use of repeated cold stress for reducing fatigue in chronic fatigue syndrome: a hypothesis. *Behavioral and Brain Functions, 3*, 1–6.

Shevchuk, N. A. (2008). Hydrotherapy as a possible neuroleptic and sedative treatment. *Medical Hypotheses, 70*(2), 230–238.

Tipton, M. J. (1989). The initial responses to cold-water immersion in man. *Clinical Science, 77*(6), 581–588.

Torres-Ronda, L., & i del Alcázar, X. S. (2014). The properties of water and their applications for training. *Journal of Human Kinetics, 44*, 237–248.

van Tubergen, A., & van der Linden, S. (2002). A brief history of spa therapy. *Annals of the Rheumatic Diseases, 61*(3), 273–275.

Veldema, J., & Jansen, P. (2021). Aquatic therapy in stroke rehabilitation: systematic review and meta-analysis. *Acta Neurologica Scandinavica, 143*(3), 221–241.

Yurtkuran, M., Yurtkuran, M., Alp, A., Nasırcılar, A., Bingöl, Ü., Altan, L., & Sarpdere, G. (2006). Balneotherapy and tap water therapy in the treatment of knee osteoarthritis. *Rheumatology International, 27*, 19–27.

Chapter 2
Shifting Paradigms in Disability Perspectives

The understanding of disability has undergone substantial conceptual shifts over the past several decades, leading to the development of three dominant frameworks that shape discourse, policy, and practice: the medical model, the social model, and the affirmative model of disability. Each of these paradigms offers a distinct lens through which disability is interpreted, influencing both theoretical analysis and practical implementation in diverse fields. These paradigms offer distinct yet complementary perspectives on the causes and implications of disability, influencing societal attitudes, institutional policies, and the lived experiences of individuals with disabilities.

While the medical model conceptualises disability as an individual deficit requiring intervention, the social model highlights systemic barriers that create limited conditions, and the affirmative model reframes disability as an inherent and valuable aspect of identity and culture. Together, these models contribute to an evolving dialogue that challenges traditional assumptions and advocates for more inclusive and empowering approaches to disability. This chapter critically examines these models, tracing their theoretical foundations and evaluating their impact on inclusive practices, disability rights, and therapeutic approaches. By situating these paradigms within broader social and political contexts, the chapter aims to provide a comprehensive understanding of their significance in shaping contemporary rehabilitation and educational frameworks.

THE MEDICAL MODEL: INDIVIDUAL IMPAIRMENT AND REHABILITATION

The medical model has historically dominated healthcare, rehabilitation, and clinical practices, positioning disability as a physiological or psychological condition residing within the individual (Forrester, 2024). Emerging from a tradition of

DOI: 10.4324/9781003659709-4

scientific advancement, the model conceptualises disability primarily as a deviation from biological or psychological norms. Rooted in 19th-century medical advancements, this model emphasises diagnosis, treatment, and rehabilitation as primary means of addressing impairment, with a focus on restoring function through medical intervention. Within this framework, therapeutic success is often measured by the degree to which bodily or cognitive functions are restored or approximated to perceived norms. This perspective has driven significant advancements in assistive technologies, surgical interventions, and rehabilitation programmes, improving the quality of life for many individuals with disabilities.

Despite its contributions, the medical model has faced extensive criticism for its narrow, deficit-based perspective. Scholars argue that it tends to frame disability as a problem to be fixed, reinforcing stigmatisation by implying that disability is inherently undesirable (Linton, 1998). Furthermore, this model places undue emphasis on individual adaptation while neglecting broader structural barriers that restrict participation in society (Shakespeare et al., 2009). By locating the source of disadvantage solely within the individual, the model fails to acknowledge the societal and environmental factors that shape disability experiences. Disability studies and advocacy movements have therefore emphasised the need for an expanded framework that integrates both medical and social dimensions of disability to better reflect lived experiences.

Stigma against individuals with disabilities is a critical concern within the medical model. Stigma is broadly defined as a social process that devalues individuals based on a characteristic perceived as undesirable, leading to discrimination, exclusion, and internalised negative self-perceptions (O'Connell et al., 2008; Lund, 2021). There are several types of stigma relevant to individuals with disabilities: (1) public stigma, which manifests as negative stereotypes and discrimination from society (O'Connell et al., 2008); (2) self-stigma, wherein individuals with disabilities internalise societal prejudices, leading to decreased self-worth (Lund, 2021); and (3) institutional stigma, where policies and practices within healthcare, education, and employment reinforce exclusion and inequality (Bergstrom et al., 2023; Lund, 2021). These interconnected forms of stigma are often unintentionally perpetuated by medicalised narratives that present disability as deviation and deficiency. The medical model often reinforces these forms of stigma by portraying disability as a defect in need of correction rather than as a valued aspect of human diversity.

An important critique of the medical model is its entanglement with ableism, which is the societal privileging of able-bodied norms and reinforces the assumption that disability is an inherent disadvantage rather than a valued form of human diversity (O'Connell et al., 2008). Ableist structures shape medical discourse by positioning disability as a deviation from normalcy, necessitating correction or elimination rather than accommodation and acceptance. This paradigm influences how medical professionals engage with individuals with disabilities, often reinforcing paternalistic attitudes that undermine autonomy and self-determination.

Recent critiques suggest renaming the medical model as the 'normalisation model of disability' to better reflect the systemic pressure to conform to able-bodied norms rather than simply receiving medical care (Zaks, 2024). This perspective argues that societal expectations of normalcy, rather than the medical interventions themselves, have historically marginalised individuals with disabilities (Barnes, 2018; Barton, 2018). Such critiques call for a deeper examination of cultural assumptions embedded within medical and rehabilitation practices.

It is important, however, not to conflate this critique of 'normalisation' with the original Scandinavian Normalisation Principle developed by Bank-Mikkelsen and Nirje. Their humanistic model aimed to promote equal rights, autonomy, and access to ordinary life experiences for people with disabilities. As Nirje (1969/1994) emphasised, normalisation means enabling inclusion and dignity, not enforcing conformity. The Scandinavian principle continues to inform contemporary rights-based and person-centred practices in disability services, standing in contrast to the deficit orientation of the medical model.

By shifting the focus from a purely biomedical view to a critique of normalisation, scholars emphasise that the true harm arises from cultural and institutional structures that devalue disabled bodies and minds (Barnes, 2018; Barton, 2018). This analysis invites a reconceptualisation of disability as a socially mediated experience rather than a fixed biological limitation.

While medical approaches remain essential in supporting health and function, a critical understanding of the medical model's limitations highlights the need for more inclusive, rights-based frameworks that centre autonomy, participation, and diversity in disability practice. Recognising both the contributions and the constraints of the medical model enables a more balanced, person-centred approach to rehabilitation and care.

THE SOCIAL MODEL: DISABILITY AS A SOCIAL CONSTRUCT

In contrast to the medical model, the social model of disability conceptualises disability as a socially constructed phenomenon rather than an inherent personal deficit. By reframing disability as a consequence of societal design rather than individual limitation, this paradigm fundamentally shifts the focus of intervention from the person to the environment. This paradigm asserts that individuals are disabled not by their impairments but by societal barriers, such as inaccessible infrastructure, discriminatory attitudes, and inadequate accommodations, that prevent full participation (Shakespeare et al., 2009). It emphasises societal transformation as the key to fostering accessibility and inclusion, framing disability as a natural variation of human diversity rather than a deviation from the norm (Forrester, 2024).

A defining feature of the social model is its influence on legal and policy reforms that promote inclusion. Legislative frameworks such as the Americans with Disabilities Act (ADA) (1990) in the United States, the Equality Act in the United Kingdom (2010), and the Disability Discrimination Act in Australia (1992) mark a transition from a medicalised approach to a rights-based framework that mandates accessibility and non-discrimination. These legal instruments embody the social model's emphasis on societal responsibility, establishing clear obligations to remove disabling barriers. On an international scale, the United Nations Convention on the Rights of Persons with Disabilities (CRPD) (United Nations, 2006) reinforces a commitment to ensuring equality, dignity, and societal participation, embedding the principles of the social model into global human rights discourse.

The social model directly challenges the stigma associated with disability by shifting the responsibility for exclusion away from individuals and onto societal structures (Retief & Letšosa, 2018). By identifying social attitudes and systemic barriers as the root causes of disadvantage, the model seeks to dismantle stereotypes and promote inclusive cultural norms. However, some scholars argue that while this model successfully highlights systemic discrimination, it does not fully address the psychological and social consequences of stigma, such as the internalisation of negative societal perceptions, which can contribute to mental distress and decreased self-efficacy among individuals with disabilities (Lund, 2021).

While the social model has been transformative, it has also been critiqued for its overemphasis on external barriers while downplaying the role of impairment itself in shaping individual experiences. Shakespeare (2006) argues that while the model effectively highlights systemic inequalities, it does not fully capture the complex interplay between embodiment, identity, and lived experience. This critique underscores the need for more nuanced models that recognise both the impact of social structures and the realities of impairment. This critique has led to the emergence of additional models, such as the affirmative model, which expands the discourse to include disability pride and identity.

Further critiques point out that the legal frameworks influenced by the social model, such as the ADA, sometimes unintentionally reinforce the medical model by requiring individuals with disabilities to prove their eligibility for accommodations to receive accommodations (Areheart, 2008; Bunbury, 2019). This reliance on medical certification can paradoxically sustain ableist assumptions, even within ostensibly rights-based systems. This paradox underscores the necessity of continually refining the social model to ensure it does not inadvertently sustain aspects of disability oppression. Additionally, scholars advocate for a broader understanding of disabling barriers, including economic disparity and systemic inequalities, which intersect with disability in profound ways (Berghs et al., 2019). Expanding the framework to address intersectionality offers a more comprehensive and equitable vision of social inclusion.

THE AFFIRMATIVE MODEL: DISABILITY AS A POSITIVE IDENTITY

The affirmative model of disability builds upon the social model while challenging traditional deficit-based narratives. Rather than viewing disability through the lens of tragedy or limitation, this model emphasises disability as an intrinsic and valuable aspect of identity, fostering pride, empowerment, and self-advocacy (Swain & French, 2000). Emerging from the disability rights movement and grounded in the concept of disability culture, the affirmative model promotes the recognition of disability as a natural and enriching dimension of human diversity. This paradigm rejects pity-based perspectives and instead promotes celebration of difference and positive self-identity formation.

By positioning disability as a source of identity and pride, the affirmative model offers a direct counter-narrative to stigma. It promotes disability culture, challenges ableist norms, and encourages the rejection of internalised stigma by fostering a sense of belonging and self-worth (Botha & Frost, 2020). This reorientation places emphasis on self-definition and collective solidarity within the disability community, shifting the focus from deficit to empowerment. This approach aligns with minority stress theory, which explains how discrimination and stigma contribute to distress among marginalised groups (Meyer, 2003).

Central to the affirmative model is the rejection of ableist narratives that frame disability as a deficiency. This model challenges the assumption that societal participation requires assimilation into able-bodied norms, instead advocating for the acceptance of diverse ways of moving, thinking, and engaging with the world (O'Connell et al., 2008). By embracing neurodiversity and physical diversity as natural expressions of human variation, the model seeks to dismantle exclusionary structures and cultural assumptions. By dismantling ableist biases, the affirmative model fosters a culture in which individuals with disabilities can define their experiences on their own terms rather than through a lens of limitation.

The affirmative model introduces four key orientations toward disability identity, as outlined by Darling (2003):

1.   Normalisation: The desire to lead lives similar to those without disabilities.
2.   Acquiescence: Accepting societal norms while acknowledging challenges in achieving normalisation.
3.   Crusadership: Recognising societal norms while embracing disability culture and advocating for systemic change.
4.   Affirmation: Viewing disability as a positive identity, celebrating difference, and embracing the cultural and social dimensions of disability.

Despite its empowering focus, the affirmative model has faced critiques for idealising disability identity without fully accounting for the everyday struggles and material disadvantages many individuals face. Shakespeare (2015) warns that an overemphasis on pride and celebration may obscure the reality of chronic pain, limited mobility, or social exclusion that remain part of many individuals' experiences. A nuanced application of the affirmative model thus requires acknowledging the co-existence of pride and adversity within the disability experience. While the model offers an important corrective to deficit-based views, its application in therapeutic and policy contexts must be tempered with a recognition of the challenges posed by impairments themselves. A balanced approach would therefore integrate affirmation with structural and material support, ensuring that empowerment does not rely solely on psychological reframing but is grounded in real-world accessibility and resources.

From a psychological perspective, the development of a positive disability identity is closely linked to broader theories of identity formation. Erikson's (1959) framework on identity development provides insight into how individuals navigate societal attitudes and personal experiences to construct a positive self-concept. This developmental process is particularly significant during adolescence and young adulthood, critical periods for self-definition and social integration. This process is particularly significant for adolescents and young adults with disabilities, who may face unique challenges in integrating disability into their sense of self. Research suggests that therapeutic interventions can facilitate this identity formation by providing a space for self-expression, empowerment, and self-knowing (Force, 2019).

The affirmative model aligns closely with recent calls for an 'empowerment model' of disability, which focuses on self-determination and rejecting societal attempts to define disabled experiences solely through external frameworks. This empowerment-oriented perspective prioritises individual agency, encouraging people with disabilities to articulate their own narratives and aspirations. This approach encourages individuals with disabilities to redefine their own narratives and prioritise agency over external validation (Oliver, 2018). Furthermore, scholars suggest that a shift toward an anti-normalisation stance, which values all body and brain variations without pressure to conform, could serve as a more radical extension of the affirmative model (Cameron, 2014; Clare, 2017). Such a shift would not merely accommodate diversity but actively celebrate it as central to a just and inclusive society.

IMPLICATIONS FOR THERAPY AND INCLUSIVE PRACTICES

The integration of the social and affirmative models into therapy and professional practice has far-reaching implications for fostering inclusivity and empowerment. These evolving frameworks call for a fundamental shift from deficit remediation to the affirmation of agency, identity, and social participation. Traditional therapeutic approaches that focus solely on overcoming impairments are increasingly being supplemented with interventions that emphasise self-acceptance, autonomy, and pride in disability identity. McCormack and Collins (2012) argue that incorporating the affirmative model into therapy enhances client-centred approaches by prioritising self-worth and identity validation over deficit-focused interventions.

Moreover, the expansion of disability-inclusive policies across sectors, including education, employment, and healthcare, reflects the broader impact of these evolving frameworks. Legislative and institutional reforms increasingly recognise that supporting individuals with disabilities requires dismantling structural barriers rather than merely treating impairments. As disability discourse continues to evolve, interdisciplinary approaches that combine elements of the medical, social, and affirmative models provide a comprehensive understanding of disability, ensuring that individuals receive support that aligns with their lived experiences and aspirations.

The conceptualisation of disability has evolved from a primarily medicalised understanding to one that recognises the societal and cultural dimensions of disability. While the medical model remains integral to healthcare and rehabilitation, it is increasingly complemented by the social and affirmative models, which emphasise systemic change, rights-based advocacy, and identity affirmation. This paradigm shift has profoundly influenced contemporary disability policies, inclusive practices, and therapeutic approaches, fostering environments where individuals with disabilities are empowered to define their own experiences. As research and advocacy continue to advance, the integration of these models provides a foundation for a more inclusive, equitable, and affirming society.

Building on these developments, recent contributions from critical disability studies have further deepened and complicated the theoretical landscape. Scholars propose that disability must be understood not only as a social construction or cultural identity but also as a complex interplay of embodiment, relationality, and power (Goodley, 2013; Shakespeare, 2015). Critical disability studies reject simplistic binaries such as normal/abnormal or able/disabled, and instead emphasise the dynamic entanglement between physical, psychological, and socio-structural factors. Such perspectives offer a critical realist lens that recognises both the material realities of impairment and the socially mediated experience of disability (Bhaskar & Danermark, 2006). They call for therapeutic and policy frameworks that integrate agency, identity, and systemic critique, laying the groundwork for more holistic and justice-oriented practices.

Recent perspectives highlight the importance of integrating lived experiences into therapeutic settings. Disability-affirming therapy approaches emphasise empowering individuals by validating their identities, challenging internalised stigma, and ensuring accessibility within health services (Bergstrom et al., 2023). By centring the voices and expertise of individuals with disabilities, these approaches move beyond traditional models of care towards collaborative, dignity-enhancing practices. This model aligns with broader disability justice frameworks advocating for systemic change within healthcare and social services (O'Connell et al., 2008).

Another emerging perspective highlights the importance of distinguishing between medical treatment and the broader ideology of normalisation in therapeutic settings. While medical interventions play a crucial role in addressing individual health needs, scholars argue that therapy should move beyond a focus on 'correcting' impairments and instead prioritise the well-being and self-defined goals of individuals with disabilities (Zaks, 2024). Therapeutic engagement must be reframed as a process of empowerment rather than normalisation. Additionally, scholars advocate for a justice-based approach to healthcare and therapy, recognising that many of the barriers faced by individuals with disabilities stem from broader systemic inequalities rather than intrinsic impairments. This perspective aligns with efforts to reframe therapy as a means of promoting social justice and challenging discriminatory structures, rather than solely focusing on symptom management (Meekosha & Soldatic, 2011; Pellow, 2016). Such an ethical shift calls on therapists to act not only as facilitators of recovery but also as advocates for equity, dignity, and relational engagement.

In this context, value-based rehabilitation offers a compelling framework. Inclusive rehabilitation must be guided by humanistic values such as respect, justice, interdependence, and cultural humility. These principles challenge purely biomedical approaches and encourage practitioners to centre the lived realities, agency, and identities of individuals in their care (Mpofu et al., 2010). By embedding these values into rehabilitation practice, therapists can move toward a genuinely inclusive and person-centred model.

The evolving paradigms of disability are not only theoretical; they carry profound implications for therapeutic approaches, policy frameworks, and the lived experiences of individuals. The following discussion explores how these models shape contemporary practices and lay the foundation for new, inclusive frameworks. These integrative approaches seek to create systems that are not only accessible but also empowering, responsive to the diversity of human embodiment and experience.

In line with critical realist perspectives, which seek to understand disability as a result of the interaction between physical embodiment, psychological experience, and socio-cultural structures (Bhaskar & Danermark, 2006), this book moves beyond dualistic or linear models of disability. The chapters that follow build on this integrated view to propose a new framework for hydrotherapy that is both inclusive and affirming, responsive to individual complexity, environmental barriers, and the need for systemic change. Through this lens, hydrotherapy is reimagined not merely as a clinical intervention, but as a relational, rights-based practice embedded within broader movements for social justice and inclusion.

REFERENCES

Areheart, B. A. (2008). When disability isn't just right: The entrenchment of the medical model of disability and the goldilocks dilemma. *Ind. LJ, 83*, 181–232.

Australia. (1992). *Disability Discrimination Act 1992 (Cth)*. Available at: www.legislation.gov.au/Details/C2016C00763

Barnes, C. (2018). Theories of disability and the origins of the oppression of disabled people in western society. In *Disability and Society* (pp. 43–60). Routledge.

Barton, L. (2018). Sociology and disability: Some emerging issues. In *Disability and Society* (pp. 3–17). Routledge.

Berghs, M., Atkin, K., Hatton, C., & Thomas, C. (2019). Do disabled people need a stronger social model: a social model of human rights? *Disability & Society, 34*(7–8), 1034–1039.

Bergstrom, T., Reid, B. M., Lee, S. Y., & Stroud, L. R. (2023). The history of clinical psychology and its relationship to ableism: Using the past to inform future directions in disability-affirming care. *The Behavior Therapist, 46*(7), 255–261.

Bhaskar, R., & Danermark, B. (2006). Metatheory, interdisciplinarity and disability research: A critical realist perspective. *Scandinavian Journal of Disability Research, 8*(4), 278–297.

Botha, M., & Frost, D. M. (2020). Extending the minority stress model to understand mental health problems experienced by the autistic population. *Society and Mental Health, 10*(1), 20–34.

Bunbury, S. (2019). Unconscious bias and the medical model: How the social model may hold the key to transformative thinking about disability discrimination. *International Journal of Discrimination and the Law, 19*(1), 26–47.

Cameron, C. (2014). Developing an affirmative model of disability and impairment. In J. Swain, S. French, C. Barnes, & C. Thomas (eds.), *Disabling Barriers – Enabling Environments* (3rd ed., pp. 24–30). Sage.

Clare, E. (2017). Notes on natural worlds, disabled bodies, and a politics of cure. In S. J. Ray & J. Sibara (Eds.), *Disability studies and the environmental humanities: Toward an eco-crip theory* (pp. 242–265). University of Nebraska Press

Darling, R. B. (2003). Toward a model of changing disability identities: A proposed typology and research agenda. *Disability & Society, 18*(7), 881–895.

Erikson, E. (1959). Theory of identity development. In *Identity and the Life Cycle*. Nueva York: International Universities Press.

Forrester, D. (2024). The social model. In *The Enlightened Social Worker* (pp. 89–100). Policy Press.

Force, V. (2019). Art therapy as a tool for enhancing adolescent identity formation, self-knowing, and empowerment (Master's capstone thesis, Lesley University). DigitalCommons@Lesley.

Goodley, D. (2013). Dis/entangling critical disability studies. *Disability & Society, 28*(5), 631–644.

Linton, S. (1998). *Claiming Disability: Knowledge and Identity*. New York University Press.

Lund, E. M. (2021). Examining the potential applicability of the minority stress model for explaining suicidality in individuals with disabilities. *Rehabilitation Psychology, 66*(2), 183–191.

McCormack, C., & Collins, B. (2012). The affirmative model of disability: A means to include disability orientation in occupational therapy? *British Journal of Occupational Therapy, 75*(3), 156–158.

Meekosha, H., & Soldatic, K. (2011). Human rights and the global South: The case of disability. *Third World Quarterly, 32*(8), 1383–1397.

Meyer, I. H. (2003). Prejudice, social stress, and mental health in lesbian, gay, and bisexual populations: Conceptual issues and research evidence. *Psychological Bulletin, 129*(5), 674–697.

Mpofu, E., Bishop, M., Hirschi, A., & Hawkins, T. (2010). Assessment of values. In E. Mpofu & T. Oakland (eds), *Rehabilitation and Health Assessment: Applying ICF Guidelines* (pp. 381–398). Springer Publishing Company.

Nirje, B. (1994). The normalization principle and its human management implications. *SRV-VRS: The International Social Role Valorization Journal, 1*(2), 19–23. (Original work published 1969).

Pellow, D. N. (2016). Toward a critical environmental justice studies: Black Lives Matter as an environmental justice challenge. *Du Bois Review: Social Science Research on Race*, *13*(2), 221–236.

Retief, M., & Letšosa, R. (2018). Models of disability: A brief overview. *HTS Teologiese Studies/ Theological Studies*, *74*(1), a4738.

Shakespeare, T. (2006). The social model of disability. In *The Disability Studies Reader* (2nd edn, pp. 197–204). Routledge.

Shakespeare, T. (2015). *Disability Research Today*. Routledge.

Shakespeare, T., Iezzoni, L. I., & Groce, N. E. (2009). Disability and the training of health professionals. *The Lancet*, *374*(9704), 1815–1816.

Swain, J., & French, S. (2000). Towards an affirmation model of disability. *Disability & Society*, *15*(4), 569–582.

O'Connell, C., Finnerty, J., & Egan, O. (2008). *Hidden Voices: An Exploratory Study of Young Carers in Cork*. Combat Poverty Agency.

Oliver, M. (2018). A sociology of disability or a disablist sociology? In *Disability and Society* (pp. 18–42). Routledge.

United Kingdom. (2010). *Equality Act 2010*. Available at: www.legislation.gov.uk/ukpga/2010/15/contents

United Nations. (2006). *Convention on the Rights of Persons with Disabilities*. Available at: www.un.org/development/desa/disabilities/convention-on-the-rights-of-persons-with-disabilities.html

United States. (1990). *Americans with Disabilities Act of 1990, 42 U.S.C. § 12101 et seq*. Available at: www.ada.gov/

Zaks, Z. (2024). Changing the medical model of disability to the normalization model of disability: Clarifying the past to create a new future direction. *Disability & Society*, *39*(12), 3233–3260.

Chapter 3
From Medical Reductionism to Inclusive and Affirmative Hydrotherapy Frameworks

LIMITATIONS OF THE MEDICAL MODEL IN HYDROTHERAPY

The traditional medical model in healthcare has long been critiqued for its narrow, disease-centric focus. Rooted in a biomedical paradigm, this framework views health primarily through the lens of pathology and impairment. This framework emphasises diagnosing and treating impairments as isolated, individual problems, often overlooking the broader social, psychological, and environmental factors that contribute to health and well-being (World Health Organization, 2022). Hydrotherapy, with its potential to offer both physical and psychosocial benefits, exemplifies the limitations of this approach. When treatment is centred exclusively on physical recovery metrics, traditional hydrotherapy programmes risk underutilising the multidimensional therapeutic potential inherent in water-based interventions.

A central limitation of the medical model is its deficit-based perspective, which prioritises 'fixing' impairments rather than recognising disability as an integral aspect of human diversity. This framing not only medicalises disability but also constrains the scope of therapeutic goals, reinforcing limited notions of success and recovery. This approach can contribute to stigmatisation, reinforcing ableist attitudes that frame disability as a condition requiring correction rather than adaptation and inclusion (World Health Organization, 2022). For instance, a hydrotherapy programme or study designed for individuals with cerebral palsy may focus primarily on improving muscle tone, range of motion, strength, walking ability, or neuromuscular coordination (Abdelaal & Atia, 2023; Getz et al., 2012; Lee et al., 2014; Thabet et al., 2017; Wenwen, 2018; Xiang et al., 2024), while overlooking

DOI: 10.4324/9781003659709-5

the equally significant social and emotional benefits of hydrotherapy, such as fostering independence, self-efficacy, peer interaction, and quality of life (Colver et al., 2015; Garcia et al., 2012; Muñoz-Blanco et al., 2020). Such omissions limit the transformative potential of hydrotherapy to promote holistic well-being and inclusive participation.

APPLYING THE SOCIAL MODEL TO HYDROTHERAPY

The social model of disability shifts the focus from individual impairments to the societal and environmental barriers that restrict participation. Rather than perceiving disability as a personal tragedy, this model frames exclusion as a failure of societal structures to accommodate human diversity. It advocates for structural and attitudinal changes that enable individuals with disabilities to access and benefit from therapeutic interventions on equal terms (Shakespeare et al., 2009). In the context of hydrotherapy, this perspective calls for an emphasis on accessibility, adaptive equipment, and inclusive programme design to ensure meaningful engagement for all individuals, regardless of physical ability.

A clear example of the social model's application in hydrotherapy is the Halliwick Concept, which was originally developed to teach individuals with disabilities to swim and move independently in water (Lambeck & Gamper, 2011). Rather than aiming to correct impairments, this approach emphasises environmental adaptation, the removal of physical barriers, and the fostering of ability rather than limitation. Conducted in a group setting, the Halliwick Concept promotes social inclusion and confidence, encouraging peer support and collective participation, which enhance both physical and emotional well-being (Garcia et al., 2012). By centring the environment rather than the individual's perceived limitations, the Halliwick Concept exemplifies the transformative potential of socially inclusive aquatic practices.

Despite the promise of such inclusive models, significant structural and social barriers continue to limit participation in hydrotherapy. Many facilities lack appropriate infrastructure, such as ramps, lifts, and designated changing areas, thereby deterring individuals with disabilities from engaging in aquatic therapy (Pourghane, 2017; Rimmer et al., 2005; Rimmer et al., 2017). Physical inaccessibility remains a major obstacle to full participation, reflecting systemic neglect of diverse access needs. Moreover, prevailing misconceptions about disability further restrict participation in physical activity programmes (Shields & Synnot, 2016). Such attitudes perpetuate exclusion by positioning disability as incompatible with active engagement and therapeutic benefit.

In contrast, some community-based aquatic programmes such as the Arthritis Foundation Aquatic Program (AFAP) offer promising examples of inclusive practice. AFAP's group format, broad accessibility, and integration into community settings reflect core principles of the social model, including the removal of participation barriers and the promotion of social connection and belonging (Cadmus et al., 2010). By embedding hydrotherapy within familiar, accessible environments, these initiatives foster continuity between therapy and everyday community life. These qualities are essential for individuals who may otherwise experience isolation due to disability-related challenges.

However, inclusive hydrotherapy is not only a matter of physical access. A lack of disability competency among healthcare professionals can result in programmes that unintentionally exclude individuals with specific needs (Marjadi et al., 2023). For instance, hydrotherapy sessions that do not provide tactile markers, auditory cues, or structured orientation strategies may be inaccessible to individuals with visual impairments (Nissim et al., 2022). Without such adaptations, hydrotherapy risks becoming an exclusionary rather than inclusive practice. True inclusivity demands not only environmental adaptation but also attitudinal and procedural shifts among practitioners.

Beyond the poolside environment, systemic inequities in healthcare settings compound these challenges. Research has shown that healthcare providers' limited awareness of disability-inclusive care contributes to ongoing barriers to participation and to health inequities more broadly (Marjadi et al., 2023). Stereotypes and assumptions about disability can further result in therapeutic approaches that ignore participants' goals and preferences, thereby undermining person-centred care. Such practices reinforce medical paternalism, limiting the autonomy and agency of individuals seeking rehabilitation.

To address these challenges, inclusive training for hydrotherapy professionals is essential. Clinicians must receive education that fosters a strength-based understanding of disability, as well as practical skills for adapting communication and physical environments. This includes improving access through alternative formats, signage, and pool entry systems. Training must also promote cultural humility and an openness to diverse ways of engaging in therapeutic activities.

Finally, systemic advocacy is critical. Providers and institutions must work toward policy reforms that embed accessibility, autonomy, and equity within hydrotherapy practices. Advocacy efforts should extend beyond individual facilities to address structural inequities across health and rehabilitation systems. By embedding the social model within hydrotherapy, professionals can move beyond a narrow rehabilitative focus and towards a holistic and empowering approach that acknowledges disability as part of human diversity. Such a shift reframes hydrotherapy as a platform for social participation, dignity, and self-determination.

AFFIRMATIVE MODEL: EMPOWERMENT THROUGH HYDROTHERAPY

Building upon the social model's emphasis on removing barriers, the affirmative model further shifts the focus toward empowerment, identity, and active participation. Rather than viewing disability solely as a challenge requiring accommodation, this model celebrates it as an integral and valuable aspect of human diversity (Swain & French, 2000). The affirmative model moves beyond a paradigm of access to one of agency and flourishing, positioning disability not as a limitation but as a positive dimension of selfhood. It moves beyond inclusion to actively promote autonomy, self-determination, and confidence, ensuring that individuals with disabilities are not merely accommodated in hydrotherapy programmes but are recognised as equal participants with agency in their own therapeutic process.

In hydrotherapy, the affirmative model transforms the therapeutic experience by prioritising self-efficacy, personal choice, and emotional well-being. Traditional rehabilitation frameworks often focus on functional improvements such as muscle strength and balance (Esmailiyan et al., 2023; Kim et al., 2020). While these aspects remain valuable, the affirmative model encourages a more holistic approach, recognising that hydrotherapy also plays a critical role in fostering confidence, self-esteem, and a positive self-identity. Therapeutic success is thus measured not only by biomechanical outcomes but also by the extent to which individuals feel empowered, connected, and affirmed.

One practical application of this model is the Water World Swimming Therapy method, developed by Ori Sela, which tailors swimming techniques to individual physical structures and needs, ensuring that movements are adapted rather than standardised. By focusing on personal strengths rather than limitations, Water World Swimming Therapy encourages individuals to engage with the water in a way that suits their unique abilities, fostering a sense of self-efficacy and autonomy. Additionally, Water World Swimming Therapy is often practised in group settings, creating a supportive and socially engaging environment where individuals benefit from shared experiences, mutual encouragement, and collective participation. *This community-based dimension reinforces emotional resilience and nurtures a sense of belonging, integral components of psychological well-being.*

Beyond its physical benefits, hydrotherapy has been shown to enhance self-esteem, emotional regulation, and overall psychological resilience. Research suggests that warm water immersion (33.5–35.5°C) elicits a relaxation response by increasing parasympathetic nervous system activity, leading to reduced stress levels and improved perceived well-being (Carere & Orr, 2016). The sensory richness of the aquatic environment, combined with buoyancy that reduces gravitational constraints, enables individuals to experience a sense of ease, safety, and mastery over movement. The calming effect of water creates an environment where individuals feel more at ease and in control of their movements, which can be particularly empowering for those who experience mobility restrictions on land.

Hydrotherapy has also demonstrated positive effects on confidence in children with autism spectrum disorders (ASD). Studies indicate that structured aquatic therapy programmes can enhance social engagement, peer interaction, and emotional regulation, contributing to greater independence and self-confidence (Pan, 2010; Chu & Pan, 2012). These findings reinforce the affirmative model's emphasis on identity development and empowerment, illustrating how hydrotherapy fosters social and emotional growth alongside physical benefits.

The transition from hydrotherapy to adaptive aquatic sports, including Paralympic swimming, exemplifies how the affirmative model fosters self-determination, confidence, and identity formation. Participation in sport provides individuals with disabilities opportunities to develop physical competence, redefine personal abilities, and gain a sense of mastery over their movements, reinforcing the concept of disability as a source of strength rather than limitation (Jefferies et al., 2012). Adaptive sports thus represent a continuum of empowerment that begins with therapeutic engagement and extends into self-directed achievement and community participation.

Many Paralympic swimmers begin their journey in therapeutic aquatic environments, using hydrotherapy as an entry point into structured training, competitive sport, and self-actualisation. Adaptive swimming programmes and community-based aquatic initiatives build upon the foundation of buoyancy-supported movement, water-based strength training, and neuromuscular coordination, offering individuals a pathway to progress beyond rehabilitation toward long-term physical and psychological empowerment. Research highlights that athletic participation in adaptive sports enhances self-perception, social identity, and resilience, with athletes frequently reporting increased self-confidence, personal independence, and a stronger sense of community belonging (Banack et al., 2011; Wheeler et al., 1999). Such trajectories illustrate how hydrotherapy, when informed by an affirmative perspective, can catalyse enduring positive identity development and social engagement.

By shifting the focus from impairment to empowerment, the affirmative model reframes hydrotherapy as an opportunity for individuals with disabilities to explore their strengths, build resilience, and cultivate a sense of autonomy. While rehabilitation remains an essential goal, the affirmative model expands the purpose of hydrotherapy to include personal growth, self-expression, and identity affirmation. This perspective challenges deficit-based narratives, positioning hydrotherapy not merely as a means of functional recovery but as a relational, rights-based practice that honours individual agency and fosters full participation in society.

THE INTERNATIONAL CLASSIFICATION OF FUNCTIONING, DISABILITY AND HEALTH (ICF) FRAMEWORK: BRIDGING FUNCTIONING AND CONTEXT

The International Classification of Functioning, Disability and Health (ICF) provides a biopsychosocial framework that integrates both medical and social perspectives on health and disability. By conceptualising disability as the result of dynamic interactions between health conditions and contextual factors, the ICF moves beyond purely biomedical models. It categorises functioning and disability into three primary components: body functions and structures, activities and participation, and contextual factors, including environmental and personal attributes (World Health Organization, 2001). By considering the interaction between these components, the ICF offers a comprehensive approach to assessing participation in hydrotherapy.

Recent research highlights the utility of the ICF framework in identifying participation restrictions and environmental facilitators in hydrotherapy for children with disabilities (Hadar-Frumer et al., 2023). This study emphasises the role of aquatic environments not only as therapeutic spaces but also as contexts that can either enable or restrict participation. By providing a structured lens for evaluating environmental and personal factors, the ICF supports the development of interventions that promote accessibility, equity, and inclusion. The structured approach of the ICF allows practitioners to systematically evaluate these contextual factors, ensuring that hydrotherapy interventions promote inclusion and accessibility.

However, while the ICF acknowledges environmental and personal factors, it does not explicitly incorporate identity formation and empowerment, which are central to the affirmative model. This omission limits the framework's ability to fully capture the transformative dimensions of rehabilitation that relate to self-efficacy, pride, and disability identity. This limitation restricts its ability to fully capture the transformative potential of hydrotherapy in fostering disability pride and self-determination.

The limitations of the ICF in addressing empowerment and identity have implications for both practice and research. Expanding the ICF to include affirmative dimensions could enable researchers to assess not only functional outcomes but also the ways in which individuals perceive and embrace their identities through therapeutic processes. Such an expansion would offer a more holistic understanding of rehabilitation outcomes, reflecting both functional and psychosocial domains. While adaptations of the ICF, such as the ICF-CY (Children and Youth) and ICF-Rehabilitation, offer more targeted approaches, they still lack explicit integration of empowerment and identity-related dimensions in hydrotherapy.

Some scholars have called for value-based rehabilitation approaches that incorporate shared decision-making, self-advocacy, and culturally responsive care (Mpofu & Oakland, 2010). These perspectives emphasise that effective rehabilitation must go beyond functioning to support dignity, agency, and the individual's right to shape their own therapeutic journey. Such approaches align closely with rights-based and person-centred care models, offering pathways to more equitable and affirming rehabilitation practices.

Thus, the evolution of hydrotherapy requires a model that integrates body functioning, identity, social belonging, and holistic well-being, elements that are fully realised in the Four-Dimensional Model of Hydrotherapy. This comprehensive framework seeks to bridge existing gaps by recognising the interconnectedness of physical, psychological, and social dimensions within therapeutic practice. The next chapter introduces this model as a structured, holistic framework that moves beyond traditional paradigms to enhance autonomy, resilience, and inclusive participation.

REFERENCES

Abdelaal, A. A. M., & Atia, D. (2023). Efficacy of aquatic exercise on pulmonary function and aquatic skills performance in older children with cerebral palsy. Randomised controlled study. *Physiotherapy Quarterly, 31*(4), 81–86.

Banack, H. R., Sabiston, C. M., & Bloom, G. A. (2011). Coach autonomy support, basic need satisfaction, and intrinsic motivation of paralympic athletes. *Research Quarterly for Exercise and Sport, 82*(4), 722–730.

Cadmus, L., Patrick, M. B., Maciejewski, M. L., Topolski, T. A. R. I., Belza, B. A. S. I. A., & Patrick, D. L. (2010). Community-based aquatic exercise and quality of life in persons with osteoarthritis. *Medicine & Science in Sports & Exercise*, *42*(1), 8–15.

Carere, M., & Orr, R. (2016). Hydrotherapy: Applications in stress reduction and wellness. *Journal of Aquatic Therapy*, *8*(2), 12–19.

Chu, C. H., & Pan, C. Y. (2012). The effect of aquatic programs on children with autism spectrum disorders: A systematic review. *Research in Autism Spectrum Disorders*, *6*(3), 993–1002.

Colver, A., Rapp, M., Eisemann, N., Ehlinger, V., Thyen, U., Dickinson, H. O., Jackie Parkes, J., Kathryn Parkinson, K., Nystrand, M., Fauconnier, J., Marcelli, M., Michelsen, S. I., & Arnaud, C. (2015). Self-reported quality of life of adolescents with cerebral palsy: A cross-sectional and longitudinal analysis. *The Lancet*, *385*(9969), 705–716.

Esmailiyan, M., Marandi, S. M., Darvishi, M., Javanmard, S. H., & Amerizadeh, A. (2023). The effect of eight weeks of aquatic exercises on muscle strength in children with cerebral palsy: A case study. *Advanced Biomedical Research*, *12*(1), 87–94.

Garcia, M. K., Joares, E. C., Silva, M. A., Bissolotti, R. R., Oliveira, S., & Battistella, L. R. (2012). The Halliwick Concept, inclusion and participation through aquatic functional activities. *Acta Fisiatr*, *12*(3), 142–150.

Getz, M., Hutzler, Y., Vermeer, A., Yarom, Y., & Unnithan, V. (2012). The effect of aquatic and land-based training on the metabolic cost of walking and motor performance in children with cerebral palsy: a pilot study. *International Scholarly Research Notices*, *2012*(1), 657979.

Hadar-Frumer, M., Ben-Shabat, E., & Weiss, P. L. (2023). Using the International Classification of Functioning, Disability and Health (ICF) to assess hydrotherapy participation for children with disabilities. *Disability and Rehabilitation*, 45(5), 789–797.

Jefferies, P., Gallagher, P., & Dunne, S. (2012). The Paralympic athlete: a systematic review of the psychosocial literature. *Prosthetics and Orthotics International*, *36*(3), 278–289.

Kim, Y., Vakula, M. N., Waller, B., & Bressel, E. (2020). A systematic review and meta-analysis comparing the effect of aquatic and land exercise on dynamic balance in older adults. *BMC Geriatrics*, *20*, 1–14.

Lambeck, J., & Gamper, U. N. (2011). The Halliwick concept. In J. Lambeck & U. Gamper (eds), *Comprehensive Aquatic Therapy* (3rd edn). Washington State University Publishing.

Lee, H. Y., Cha, Y. J., & Kim, K. (2014). The effect of feedback respiratory training on pulmonary function of children with cerebral palsy: A randomized controlled preliminary report. *Clinical Rehabilitation*, *28*(10), 965–971.

Marjadi, B., Flavel, J., Baker, K., Glenister, K., Morns, M., Triantafyllou, M., Strauss, P., Wolff, B., Procter, A. M., Mengesha, Z., Walsberger, S., Qiao, X., & Gardiner, P. A. (2023). Twelve tips for inclusive practice in healthcare settings. *International Journal of Environmental Research and Public Health*, *20*(5), 4657.

Mpofu, E., & Oakland, T. (2010). *Rehabilitation and Health Assessment: Applying ICF Guidelines*. Springer.

Muñoz-Blanco, E., Merino-Andrés, J., Aguilar-Soto, B., García, Y. C., Puente-Villalba, M., Pérez-Corrales, J., & Güeita-Rodríguez, J. (2020). Influence of aquatic therapy in children and youth with cerebral palsy: A qualitative case study in a special education school. *International Journal of Environmental Research and Public Health*, *17*(10), 3690.

Nissim, M., Ariel N., & Alter, E. (2022). Practical applications of aquatic physical activity, swimming, and therapy for people with visual impairment or blindness. *Movement*, *13*(3), 1–17.

Pan, C. Y. (2010). The effect of aquatic intervention on improving social interactions and behaviors in children with autism spectrum disorders. *Research in Autism Spectrum Disorders*, *4*(4), 477–485.

Pourghane, P. (2017). Barriers to participating in hydrotherapy in older women: A qualitative study. *Journal of Nursing and Midwifery Sciences*, *4*(1), 14–20.

Rimmer, J. H., Padalabalanarayanan, S., Malone, L. A., & Mehta, T. (2017). Fitness facilities still lack accessibility for people with disabilities. *Disability and Health Journal*, *10*(2), 214–221.

Rimmer, J. H., Riley, B., Wang, E., & Rauworth, A. (2005). Accessibility of health clubs for people with mobility disabilities and visual impairments. *American Journal of Public Health*, *95*(11), 2022–2028.

Shakespeare, T., Iezzoni, L. I., & Groce, N. E. (2009). Disability and the training of health professionals. *The Lancet*, *374*(9704), 1815–1816.

Shields, N., & Synnot, A. (2016). Perceived barriers and facilitators to participation in physical activity for children with disability: a qualitative study. *BMC Pediatrics*, *16*, 1–10.

Swain, J., & French, S. (2000). Towards an affirmation model of disability. *Disability & Society*, *15*(4), 569–582.

Thabet, N. S., Zaky, N. A., & Banoub, M. B. (2017). Underwater exercises versus treadmill training on gait in children with spastic hemiparetic cerebral palsy. *Int J Physiother Res*, *5*(5), 2385–2391.

Wenwen, L. (2018). Analysis of the effect of functional hydrotherapy on muscle strength and motor function in children with spastic cerebral palsy. *Chin J Conval Med*, *27*, 909–911.

Wheeler, G. D., Steadward, R. D., Legg, D., Hutzler, Y., Campbell, E., & Johnson, A. (1999). Personal investment in disability sport careers: An international study. *Adapted Physical Activity Quarterly*, *16*(3), 219–237.

World Health Organization. (2001). *International Classification of Functioning, Disability and Health (ICF)*. World Health Organization.

World Health Organization. (2022). *Global Perspectives on Disability and Rehabilitation: A Review of Frameworks and Policies*. World Health Organization.

Xiang, A., Fu, Y., Wang, C., Huang, D., Qi, J., Zhao, R., Wu, L., Fan, C., & Zhang, Q. (2024). Aquatic therapy for spastic cerebral palsy: A scoping review. *European Journal of Medical Research*, *29*(1), 569–575.

Part II
Core Framework
The Four-Dimensional Model

Chapter 4

Holistic Four-Dimensional Model for Hydrotherapy

Hydrotherapy is more than a collection of techniques for physical rehabilitation; it is a multifaceted, immersive environment with the potential to transform how we understand and facilitate therapeutic change. Rather than being limited to biomechanical correction, hydrotherapy offers a rich, sensory and relational context that can foster profound personal growth and social engagement. Drawing on interdisciplinary insights from rehabilitation science, disability studies, psychology, and social inclusion, the Four-Dimensional Model of Hydrotherapy offers a comprehensive framework that captures the physical, emotional, social, and long-term impacts of water-based interventions.

Each dimension: Body Functioning and Sensory Experience, Affirmative Identity and Self-Determination, Social Belonging and Inclusion, and Holistic Well-Being and Long-Term Impact, builds upon the others in a dynamic, interconnected process. This integrative structure reflects the complex interplay between body, mind, and environment, recognising that therapeutic outcomes are not isolated but mutually reinforcing. Rather than presenting discrete stages, the model is conceived as a spiral of growth, where improvements in one domain create momentum for positive change in others. Progress is understood as iterative and cumulative, with each therapeutic gain opening new possibilities for further development across multiple life domains.

This structure enables practitioners and researchers alike to assess, plan, and evaluate hydrotherapy in a manner that is both evidence-informed and person-centred. By offering a multidimensional framework, the model supports interventions that are tailored to the aspirations, identities, and lived realities of individuals, moving beyond reductionist approaches. A summary Table of the Four-Dimensional Model of Hydrotherapy is presented in Table 4.1.

DOI: 10.4324/9781003659709-7

Table 4.1 Summary Table of The Four-Dimensional Model of Hydrotherapy

Dimension	Conceptual Overview	Examples for Outcome* Indicators
1. Body Functioning and Sensory Experience	This dimension addresses the motor, sensory, and pain-relief benefits of hydrotherapy.	1a. Motor: This subdimension focuses on movement capacities supported by aquatic therapy, including strength, coordination, and postural control. It recognises that goals may involve improvement, maintenance, or prevention of deterioration. 1b. Sensory: This subdimension focuses on proprioceptive, vestibular, and tactile processing, sensory modulation, and integration. Outcomes may include enhanced sensory regulation, stabilisation of sensory responses, or prevention of sensory overload. 1c. Pain: This subdimension focuses on the role of hydrotherapy in modulating pain perception and supporting comfort through thermal, hydrostatic, and proprioceptive properties of water. Outcomes may include reduced pain intensity, improved pain tolerance, stabilisation of chronic pain symptoms, or prevention of functional decline related to pain.

Dimension	Conceptual Overview	Examples for Outcome* Indicators
2. Affirmative Identity and Self-Determination	This dimension addresses the psychosocial, emotional, and identity-related benefits of hydrotherapy.	2a. Self-efficacy: This subdimension focuses on the individual's belief in their capacity to act effectively and achieve meaningful goals. Hydrotherapy may contribute to preservation of existing levels of self-efficacy, or prevention of decline in perceived competence.
		2b. Emotional regulation: This subdimension addresses the individual's ability to manage and respond to emotional experiences in adaptive ways. Outcomes may include enhanced emotional stability, improved coping with stress, or the maintenance of emotional well-being in the face of physical or psychological challenges.
		2c. Autonomy and functional independence: This subdimension highlights opportunities within hydrotherapy to support autonomous decision-making. Outcomes may include increased functional independence, preservation of self-directed participation, or prevention of over-reliance on others in care routines.
		2d. Resilience: This subdimension refers to the capacity to adapt positively in the face of adversity. Hydrotherapy may support the development or maintenance of psychological resilience by offering affirming experiences.
		2e. Stress response: This subdimension considers the role of hydrotherapy in modulating physiological and psychological responses to stress. Outcomes may include reduced stress reactivity, stabilisation of stress-related symptoms, or prevention of stress-related deterioration in health and well-being.

(Continued)

Table 4.1 (Continued)

Dimension	Conceptual Overview	Examples for Outcome* Indicators
		2f. Shared decision-making and advocacy: This subdimension recognises the importance of the individual's voice in shaping their therapeutic experience. It includes practices that enable shared decision-making, co-creation of goals, and opportunities for self-advocacy. Outcomes may include increased participation in planning sessions, enhanced ability to articulate needs and preferences, or prevention of exclusion from key decisions in care.
3. Social Belonging and Inclusion	This dimension addresses the relational, participatory, and community-oriented aspects of hydrotherapy. It emphasises the potential of aquatic settings to promote inclusive social engagement, foster a sense of belonging, and reduce barriers to interpersonal and group participation. Social inclusion is explored through multiple interrelated layers, ranging from behavioural engagement and interpersonal cooperation to subjective belonging and structural equity.	3a. Social participation (Behavioural level): This subdimension focuses on the individual's ability to engage in social, recreational. Outcomes may include increased participation in group activities, maintenance of social engagement, or prevention of social withdrawal and isolation. 3b. Group cooperation (Interpersonal level): This subdimension explores how hydrotherapy promotes collaborative interaction, mutual support, and shared goal-setting among participants. Outcomes may include enhanced interpersonal communication, sustained group involvement, or prevention of disengagement from collective therapeutic efforts. 3c. Belonging (Subjective level): This subdimension refers to the individual's experience of inclusion, emotional safety, and being valued within a group. Outcomes may include strengthened identification with a peer group, stabilisation of perceived social connectedness, or prevention of exclusion and marginalisation.

Dimension	Conceptual Overview	Examples for Outcome* Indicators
		3d. Equality (Structural level): This subdimension considers how hydrotherapy environments can foster equity by reducing physical and social hierarchies. Outcomes may include increased perceptions of mutual respect, sustained egalitarian participation, or prevention of exclusion due to functional differences.
4. Holistic Well-Being and Long-Term Impact	This dimension addresses the long-term effects of hydrotherapy on health, participation, and overall life experience. It highlights hydrotherapy's potential to support sustained well-being through functional carryover, improved quality of life, and the development of lifelong health behaviours.	4a. Functional transfer: This subdimension focuses on the application of skills, strategies, and physical capacities developed in hydrotherapy to everyday contexts. Outcomes may include generalisation of movement patterns, maintenance of daily functioning, or prevention of decline in participation across home, school, work, or community environments.
		4b. Quality of life: This subdimension reflects the individual's subjective experience of physical, emotional, and social well-being. Outcomes may include enhanced life satisfaction, stabilisation of perceived health, or prevention of reduced well-being due to chronic health challenges.
		4c. Health behaviour sustainability: This subdimension explores hydrotherapy's role in promoting continued physical activity, self-care practices, and motivation for wellness beyond the therapeutic setting. Outcomes may include ongoing engagement in movement, preservation of self-management strategies, or prevention of sedentary regression over time.

Note: *Outcome indicators may vary depending on individual goals and contextual factors such as diagnosis, age, or sensory profile.

DIMENSION 1: BODY FUNCTIONING AND SENSORY EXPERIENCE

Hydrotherapy, through the distinctive physical properties of water, has been shown to support motor performance, sensory processing, and pain management. The aquatic environment creates conditions that are uniquely conducive to functional movement and sensory regulation, offering therapeutic possibilities beyond those available in land-based rehabilitation. The buoyancy of water reduces gravitational constraints, enabling individuals to engage in movements that may be difficult or impossible on land (Becker, 2009). Hydrostatic pressure and viscosity provide consistent, evenly distributed sensory input (Sato et al., 2012), enhancing proprioceptive awareness and postural control. Additionally, the thermal properties of water contribute to muscle relaxation, improved circulation, and reduced pain perception (Prabhu & Dadmi, 2019).

Hydrotherapy has demonstrated positive effects on various aspects of motor function, such as range of motion (ROM), joint stability, postural control, and both gross and fine motor skills (Assar et al., 2020; Jain et al., 2022; Jeon et al., 2023; Kargarfard et al., 2013). The buoyancy inherent to water reduces gravitational load, facilitating movement and increasing joint flexibility. A scoping review highlighted that aquatic therapy can enhance ROM and muscle strength in individuals with spastic cerebral palsy (CP), attributing these outcomes to the unique properties of the aquatic environment (Xiang et al., 2024). Such findings reinforce the role of water-based interventions in addressing both primary impairments and secondary functional limitations.

Hydrostatic pressure and water resistance further provide a stabilising and supportive setting for improving postural control and joint function. A systematic review reported that aquatic interventions yielded significant motor benefits in children with CP, with 64% of studies documenting meaningful improvements (Mujawar, 2022). The Halliwick Concept, which emphasises core stability and dynamic balance through water-based movement, has shown particular promise in enhancing gross mobility and balance among children with CP (Chandolias et al., 2022). Moreover, systematic evidence supports the effectiveness of aquatic therapy in fostering both gross and fine motor development, underscoring its relevance across a wide range of motor rehabilitation goals (Mujawar, 2022).

Water provides an enriched sensory environment that supports enhanced body awareness and functional engagement. The hydrostatic pressure and resistance of water deliver full-body, multi-modal sensory input (proprioceptive, vestibular, tactile, and auditory) contributing to improved sensory modulation and stability. Aquatic settings thus offer a uniquely integrative sensory experience that fosters adaptive responses across multiple systems.

Aquatic interventions have been shown to be particularly effective for children on the autism spectrum. In a quasi-experimental study involving 56 children aged five to eight, a six-month structured aquatic programme led to statistically significant improvements in sensory processing, as measured by the Short Sensory Profile (Quraishi & Jarrar, 2018). Fitzpatrick (2021) further emphasised that aquatic occupational therapy offers a unique sensory experience not easily replicated in land-based settings. Water-based environments are especially conducive to sensory integration for individuals with diverse sensory processing profiles. Seven occupational therapists highlighted the potential of aquatic settings to facilitate proprioceptive and vestibular integration more effectively than conventional therapeutic environments, positioning hydrotherapy as an optimal intervention for individuals with high sensory needs or aversions. These findings suggest that aquatic environments provide both a nurturing and dynamic context for addressing sensory processing challenges.

Hydrotherapy has shown substantial benefits in pain management across various populations. For individuals with chronic low back pain, a systematic review and meta-analysis of 13 randomised controlled trials reported a large effect size in favour of hydrotherapy over no intervention (Ma et al., 2022). Furthermore, aquatic therapy was found to be more effective than land-based exercise in alleviating overall pain. This superior effect is attributed to the unique mechanical and thermal properties of water, which simultaneously modulate multiple physiological systems involved in pain perception.

Evidence also supports the role of hydrotherapy in reducing pain associated with fibromyalgia syndrome (FMS). A review of clinical studies revealed that 94% reported pain reduction following aquatic interventions (Zamunér et al., 2019). The analgesic effects are attributed to water's combined properties (buoyancy, hydrostatic pressure, thermal conduction, and resistance) which influence physiological systems including neuromuscular, cardiovascular, endocrine, and inflammatory responses. Warm water immersion promotes muscle relaxation, enhances circulation, and modulates nociceptive processing, contributing to increased pain thresholds and reduced allodynia.

As a multi-sensory intervention, hydrotherapy provides a comforting and enabling environment for movement. It is widely regarded as a non-pharmacological strategy that promotes functional mobility and well-being, particularly for individuals living with chronic pain. By offering a safe, supportive, and enriching environment, hydrotherapy supports both symptom relief and functional empowerment, reinforcing its value within a holistic rehabilitation framework.

DIMENSION 2: AFFIRMATIVE IDENTITY AND SELF-DETERMINATION

This dimension integrates insights from the affirmative model of disability (Swain and French, 2000), self-determination theory (Deci & Ryan, 2012), self-efficacy theory (Bandura, 1997), and positive psychology (Seligman & Csikszentmihalyi, 2000).

The affirmative model reframes disability not as a deficit, but as a positive and valued identity (Swain & French, 2000). Within this framework, hydrotherapy becomes a relational and empowering space in which individuals can engage with their bodies on their own terms, free from deficit-based assumptions. Rather than reinforcing a narrative of limitation, this approach affirms bodily difference as part of personal and collective identity.

Self-efficacy theory posits that mastery experiences contribute significantly to one's belief in their capabilities, reinforcing confidence and perseverance in the face of future challenges (Bandura, 1997). In hydrotherapy, the aquatic environment provides a supportive and adaptive setting in which individuals can experience success in movement, thereby strengthening their belief in their own abilities. These embodied experiences build a foundation for self-confidence and motivate ongoing participation.

Self-determination theory emphasises intrinsic motivation, autonomy, and competence as core drivers of personal growth and psychological well-being (Deci & Ryan, 2012). Hydrotherapy programmes that prioritise individual choice, collaborative goal-setting, and meaningful participation are more likely to activate these internal motivators and foster sustained engagement. When individuals are empowered to shape their therapeutic goals, the process becomes more than functional recovery – it becomes self-actualising.

Positive psychology highlights resilience, optimism, and emotional regulation as key resources for flourishing (Seligman & Csikszentmihalyi, 2000). Hydrotherapy offers individuals the opportunity to engage in empowering, affirming experiences that support psychological resilience and self-worth. These benefits extend beyond the session itself, influencing how individuals relate to their bodies and navigate the world.

Hydrotherapy provides unique opportunities to experience movement with greater fluidity and fewer physical constraints. Buoyancy reduces weight-bearing demands, allowing for movement experiences that may be difficult or impossible on land. This may contribute to a shift in self-perception, fostering bodily comfort and reinforcing a positive identity grounded not in normative physical function but in autonomy, progress, and meaningful participation.

Through repeated movement successes in the water, individuals begin to reframe their identity, not solely as someone with a limitation, but as a capable, self-directed person. This transformation is especially evident when individuals articulate a renewed relationship with their body, shifting from avoidance or frustration to curiosity, pride, or acceptance. Such internal reorientation marks a move from externally defined limitations to self-authored strength and presence. These shifts mark a fundamental transition from an externally defined disability identity to one that is internally anchored in resilience and lived bodily experience.

Emerging evidence suggests that hydrotherapy supports both physical relief and psychological empowerment. For example, a study involving women with fibromyalgia reported significant improvements in pain intensity, depressive symptoms, quality of life, and perceived self-efficacy in physical activity (Letieri et al., 2013). Similarly, an intensive aquatic Watsu programme was found to contribute to substantial improvements in emotional and behavioural self-regulation in a young adult on the autism spectrum. These improvements included enhanced tolerance of touch, reduced self-aggressive behaviours, and increased independence in daily routines, likely facilitated by the structured and sensory-rich nature of the hydrotherapy environment (Tufekcioglu et al., 2023).

The immersive nature of hydrotherapy also facilitates emotional regulation through physiological mechanisms. Immersion in warm water induces a parasympathetic response, characterised by reduced heart rate and vascular resistance, increased stroke volume, and an overall state of relaxation (Becker, 2009). Hydrostatic pressure further supports cognitive and emotional function by increasing cerebral blood flow and improving oxygen and nutrient delivery to the brain (Wilcock et al., 2006). These physiological effects create fertile ground for emotional safety, trust, and reflective engagement.

Hydrotherapy interventions have proven particularly effective in promoting functional independence among older adults. A controlled study evaluating the impact of a 12-week aquatic exercise programme using the Functional Independence Measure (FIM) found statistically significant improvements in activities of daily living, including bathing, dressing, transferring, and mobility, in comparison with a control group (Aidar et al., 2006). Another study demonstrated that an eight-month aquatic aerobic training programme significantly improved functional autonomy in older women with low bone mineral density. Participants exhibited gains in walking, sit-to-stand transfers, dressing, and overall autonomy scores (Pernambuco et al., 2013). These outcomes demonstrate the relevance of this dimension across the life course.

To fully realise hydrotherapy's potential, therapists must move beyond motor-centric goals and adopt person-centred approaches that prioritise emotional well-being, autonomy, and identity formation. This includes co-constructing goals with participants, creating opportunities for meaningful and successful movement experiences, and designing emotionally supportive, choice-driven therapeutic environments. Therapeutic relationships must be grounded in reciprocity, trust, and a shared commitment to the individual's holistic development.

Shared decision-making and self-advocacy are also central to this dimension. Person-centred hydrotherapy should not only offer opportunities for autonomy in movement but also enable individuals to shape the direction of their therapeutic journey. Co-constructing goals, inviting participants to express their preferences, and actively involving families or caregivers in planning reflect best practices in inclusive care. This approach supports the development of communicative agency and reinforces the individual's right to be an active decision-maker in their rehabilitation. Outcomes may include enhanced participation in planning sessions, improved ability to articulate therapeutic needs, and the prevention of exclusion from key decisions affecting care and progression.

When guided by inclusive values, hydrotherapy contributes to the development of a resilient and self-affirming identity. In doing so, it aligns with broader rights-based approaches to rehabilitation and offers a pathway toward emotional empowerment, personal agency, and long-term independence. This dimension reminds us that rehabilitation is not only about what the body can do, but also about how the person comes to know, trust, and value themselves through movement.

DIMENSION 3: SOCIAL BELONGING AND INCLUSION

This dimension is grounded in the social model of disability (Oliver, 2018) and participatory inclusion frameworks. It also aligns with the ICF's Activities and Participation domain, which underscores the role of interpersonal relationships, community life, and environmental facilitators in overall well-being. By focusing on the relational and structural contexts of rehabilitation, this dimension expands hydrotherapy beyond the individual to embrace collective connection and accessibility.

While the aquatic environment holds significant therapeutic potential, accessibility remains a major barrier to equal participation. Research has consistently shown that environmental factors, such as inaccessible infrastructure, inappropriate scheduling, limited staffing, and lack of adaptive equipment, can restrict individuals' ability to engage in hydrotherapy. A study identified key structural and logistical barriers to the implementation of aquatic therapy for individuals with spinal cord injury. These included the absence of ramps, inadequate changing facilities, unsuitable scheduling, and high operational costs, particularly in community-based settings (Marinho-Buzelli et al., 2019). Similarly, Rimmer, Riley, Wang and Rauworth (2005) assessed the accessibility of health and fitness facilities for people with mobility and visual impairments. Their findings revealed widespread deficiencies in advanced accessibility features such as pool lifts, zero-depth entries and properly sloped ramps, particularly in privately run centres. In a focused exploration of accessibility for individuals with visual impairments, Nissim, Ariel and Alter (2022) offered a set of comprehensive recommendations, including wide entrances, tactile floor markers, high-contrast visual cues and Braille signage, as well as programmatic adaptations such as quiet scheduling, personalised instruction and tactile learning strategies.

Collectively, these studies affirm that inclusion must begin with access, not only in social and emotional terms, but also through the elimination of architectural and systemic barriers that prevent equitable engagement. Access is not a supplementary consideration, but a foundational condition for genuine participation. Without such access, therapeutic inclusion remains aspirational rather than actualised.

The social model of disability reframes exclusion as a result of environmental and systemic barriers rather than individual impairments (Oliver, 2018). In this context, the aquatic environment offers a unique and powerful equaliser. When immersed in water, all individuals, regardless of height, posture or physical function, are positioned at eye level. This physical levelling reinforces symbolic equality and challenges ableist hierarchies that are otherwise embedded in built environments. As such, water may foster a sense of mutual recognition, shared presence and embodied inclusion.

Building on this inherent potential for equality, group-based hydrotherapy promotes teamwork, peer interaction and mutual encouragement. These sessions offer opportunities for collaborative exercises, shared goal-setting and even participant-led roles, contributing to both physical and psychosocial rehabilitation. Through these practices, hydrotherapy becomes a site of relational learning, where identity and inclusion are cultivated through movement and shared experience.

Participatory inclusion frameworks emphasise shared experience and co-constructed meaning as central to fostering connection and reducing isolation (Booth et al., 2002). Group-based formats align closely with these frameworks, encouraging relational learning and reinforcing the therapeutic value of community.

Closely related to inclusion is social belonging – the experience of feeling accepted, respected and connected within a group (Allen et al., 2022). Belonging is a fundamental human need and a critical contributor to emotional well-being, motivation and resilience (Baumeister and Leary, 1995; Allen et al., 2022). However, belonging can also be ambivalent if it is predicated on assimilation or the exclusion of others. Inclusive practice must therefore cultivate forms of belonging that affirm diversity and support authentic connection. This requires a deliberate emphasis on equity, where all participants are recognised not despite difference, but through it.

Multiple studies underscore the psychosocial value of hydrotherapy in promoting belonging. Stan (2012) highlighted the multifaceted benefits of aquatic activities for individuals with disabilities, particularly in enhancing social participation, cooperation and shared achievement. A study of children with cerebral palsy found that hydrotherapy fostered environmental engagement, communicative participation and deeper social involvement across school and family contexts (Muñoz-Blanco et al., 2020). A qualitative study examined the experiences of individuals with multiple sclerosis participating in group-based aquatic therapy. The study identified three key psychosocial outcomes: enhanced social participation, stronger environmental connection and increased social support. Participants described the aquatic environment as safe, enjoyable and empowering, citing its sensory-rich qualities and reduced physical barriers (Broach et al., 2007).

To maximise inclusion and belonging, hydrotherapy interventions should be intentionally designed to support meaningful participation across a range of abilities. This includes structuring sessions around group collaboration and cooperative challenges; encouraging peer-led roles and shared goal-setting; ensuring that physical access and environmental adaptations are in place; and fostering an emotionally safe and welcoming atmosphere. When these elements are integrated, the therapeutic process becomes not only accessible, but socially generative.

When inclusion is approached holistically, beginning with access, supported by design and realised through meaningful connection, hydrotherapy becomes not only a clinical intervention, but a space for community, identity and transformation. It becomes a place where people are seen, valued and connected through the shared experience of water.

DIMENSION 4: HOLISTIC WELL-BEING AND LONG-TERM IMPACT

This fourth dimension positions hydrotherapy not merely as a time-limited intervention, but as a catalyst for sustained health, autonomy and inclusion. Rather than viewing therapeutic outcomes as isolated to the treatment period, this perspective recognises the potential for long-term adaptation and flourishing. Gains achieved through aquatic therapy, across motor, sensory, emotional and social domains, can be internalised and generalised to daily life. When experienced holistically, hydrotherapy contributes to long-term improvements in quality of life, functional participation and psychosocial resilience.

A growing body of evidence supports hydrotherapy's long-term impact across a wide range of conditions and populations. These benefits, often maintained well beyond the intervention period, span physical, psychological and functional domains. For individuals with neurological conditions, hydrotherapy has demonstrated significant and enduring effects. A systematic review and meta-analysis of randomised controlled trials reported long-term improvements in balance among individuals with Parkinson's disease, with functional gains sustained months after intervention (Liu et al., 2023). Similarly, a randomised controlled trial employing Ai Chi-based aquatic therapy showed sustained reductions in pain and depression alongside improvements in quality of life at one-month follow-up (Pérez-de la Cruz, 2019).

In chronic health contexts, including cancer recovery, hydrotherapy also contributes to long-term adaptation. An RCT with breast cancer survivors found that an eight-week deep-water programme improved fatigue, core strength and lower-limb function, with many gains maintained at six-month follow-up (Cantarero-Villanueva et al., 2013). In a case study of a woman with treatment-resistant depression, regular cold-water immersion led to symptom reduction and discontinuation of medication over a one-year period, suggesting durable emotional and physiological effects (van Tulleken et al., 2018).

Among populations undergoing life transitions or periods of emotional vulnerability, hydrotherapy demonstrates protective psychological effects. An RCT involving pregnant women found that participation in the Supervised Water Exercise Programme significantly reduced postnatal depression scores, both immediately postpartum and at follow-up (Aguilar-Cordero et al., 2019). Such findings highlight hydrotherapy's potential to act not only as rehabilitation but also as emotional prevention and support.

In children and adolescents, long-term hydrotherapy benefits have also been documented. A multiple-case study involving children with cerebral palsy reported sustained gains in motor function, psychosocial well-being and self-perceived competence up to one year after intervention (Shelef, 2010). Similarly, children on the autism spectrum demonstrated increased swimming ability, generalised physical activity and enhanced family engagement in community routines, indicating carry-over effects into everyday life (Lawson et al., 2014).

Even within preventative health, hydrotherapy demonstrates measurable long-term effects. A prospective study found that alternating hot and cold water immersion reduced the frequency and severity of common colds over six months, suggesting adaptive immune and stress regulatory mechanisms (Ernst et al., 1990). These findings broaden hydrotherapy's relevance beyond disability contexts, positioning it within health promotion and preventative care.

Hydrotherapy also contributes to long-term self-efficacy, autonomy and emotional resilience, factors that support sustained health behaviours. The World Health Organization Disability Assessment Schedule (WHODAS 2.0) has been used to assess how therapeutic gains translate into daily function, role participation and life satisfaction. A pilot protocol aims to assess hydrotherapy's impact on neuropathic pain, functionality and quality of life in individuals with spinal cord injury, using WHODAS 2.0 and other validated tools (Campo et al., 2022). Another longitudinal randomised controlled trial will examine aquatic therapy's impact on quality of life, social participation and occupational reintegration in cancer survivors, with outcomes assessed up to 24 months post-intervention (Nissim et al., 2024).

This dimension reflects a shift from viewing hydrotherapy solely as a rehabilitative modality to recognising it as a foundation for lifelong health, inclusion and empowerment. Aquatic therapy is thus positioned not only as a means of physical recovery but as a transformative tool for constructing resilient, self-directed life trajectories. When aligned with long-term personal goals, aquatic therapy not only supports rehabilitation but fosters sustained engagement, lifestyle adaptation and ongoing socio-emotional development. In doing so, it enables individuals to extend their progress beyond the therapeutic setting, actively shaping their own health trajectories, identities and community lives.

THE ESSENTIAL ROLE OF THE FOUR-DIMENSIONAL MODEL IN HYDROTHERAPY

The Four-Dimensional Model of Hydrotherapy reframes aquatic intervention as a lifelong catalyst for transformation, rather than a time-limited clinical modality. Its four dimensions: Body Functioning and Sensory Experience, Affirmative Identity and Self-Determination, Social Belonging and Inclusion, and Holistic Well-Being and Long-Term Impact, are not linear stages, but dynamic and mutually reinforcing processes. Progress within one dimension tends to catalyse advancements in others, fostering a self-sustaining cycle of physical, emotional and social benefit. Gains in one area amplify progress in others, creating a sustained cycle of therapeutic and psychosocial benefit.

Beyond its conceptual contribution, the model offers a practical, evidence-informed framework for hydrotherapists and interdisciplinary teams. It bridges theoretical insights with everyday clinical application, providing a structure for holistic rehabilitation practice. It supports person-centred assessment, planning and evaluation, and encourages the integration of emotional, social and identity-based goals alongside physical rehabilitation. By offering shared language and measurable indicators, the model enhances collaborative practice across healthcare settings. Its flexibility ensures that it can be adapted to diverse populations and therapeutic environments, promoting consistency while allowing for individualised care.

Ultimately, the Four-Dimensional Model positions hydrotherapy not only as a means of recovery, but as a transformative, inclusive and empowering approach to long-term well-being. It enables individuals to move beyond symptom management towards resilience, participation and flourishing across the lifespan. In doing so, the model challenges reductionist views of rehabilitation and positions hydrotherapy as a relational, identity-affirming and life-enhancing process.

REFERENCES

Aguilar-Cordero, M. J., Sánchez-García, J. C., Rodriguez-Blanque, R., Sánchez-López, A. M., & Mur-Villar, N. (2019). Moderate physical activity in an aquatic environment during pregnancy (SWEP study) and its influence in preventing postpartum depression. *Journal of the American Psychiatric Nurses Association*, 25(2), 112–121.

Aidar, F. S., Reis, A. J., Carneiro, V. M., & Leite, A. M. (2006). Elderly and old adult: Aquatic physical activities and functional autonomy. *Fitness Performance Journal*, 5(5), 271–276.

Allen, K. A., Gray, D. L., Baumeister, R. F., & Leary, M. R. (2022). The need to belong: A deep dive into the origins, implications, and future of a foundational construct. *Educational Psychology Review*, 34(2), 1133–1156.

Assar, S., Gandomi, F., Mozafari, M., & Sohaili, F. (2020). The effect of Total resistance exercise vs. aquatic training on self-reported knee instability, pain, and stiffness in women with knee osteoarthritis: A randomized controlled trial. *BMC Sports Science, Medicine and Rehabilitation*, *12*, 1–13.

Bandura, A. (1997). *Self-efficacy: The Exercise of Control*. Freeman.

Baumeister, R. F., & Leary, M. R. (1995). The need to belong: Desire for interpersonal attachments as a fundamental human motivation. *Psychological Bulletin*, *117*(3), 497–529.

Becker, B. E. (2009). Aquatic therapy: Scientific foundations and clinical rehabilitation applications. *PM&R*, *1*(9), 859–872.

Booth, T., Black-Hawkins, K., & Ainscow, M. (2002). *Guía para la evaluación y mejora de la educación inclusiva*. Madrid: Consorcio Universitario para la Educación Inclusiva.

Broach, E., Dattilo, J., & McKenney, A. (2007). Effects of aquatic therapy on perceived fun or enjoyment experiences of participants with multiple sclerosis. *Therapeutic Recreation Journal*, *41*(3), 179–200.

Campo, A. R., Pacichana-Quinayáz, S. G., Bonilla-Escobar, F. J., Leiva-Pemberthy, L. M., Tovar-Sánchez, M. A., Hernández-Orobio, O. M., Arango-Hoyos, G.-P., & Mujanovic, A. (2022). Effectiveness of hydrotherapy on neuropathic pain and pain catastrophization in patients with spinal cord injury: Protocol for a pilot trial study. *JMIR Research Protocols*, *11*(4), e37255. doi:10.2196/37255.

Cantarero-Villanueva, I., Fernández-Lao, C., Cuesta-Vargas, A. I., Del Moral-Avila, R., Fernández-de-Las-Peñas, C., & Arroyo-Morales, M. (2013). The effectiveness of a deep water aquatic exercise program in cancer-related fatigue in breast cancer survivors: A randomized controlled trial. *Archives of Physical Medicine and Rehabilitation*, *94*(2), 221–230.

Chandolias, K., Zarra, E., Chalkia, A., & Hristara, A. (2022). The effect of hydrotherapy according to Halliwick concept on children with cerebral palsy and the evaluation of their balance: A randomised clinical trial. *International Journal*, *9*(4), 2349–3259.

Deci, E. L., & Ryan, R. M. (2012). Self-determination theory. *Handbook of Theories of Social Psychology*, *1*(20), 416–436.

Ernst, E., Wirz, P., & Pecho, L. (1990). Prevention of common colds by hydrotherapy: A controlled long-term prospective study. *Physiotherapy*, *76*(4), 207–210.

Fitzpatrick, C. R. (2021). The benefits of aquatic occupational therapy for children on the autism spectrum (Undergraduate honours thesis). University of Arkansas

Jain, P. P., Kanase, S. B., Rainak, A., & Kanase, S. B. (2022). Effect of aquatic exercises on postural control in elderly population. *NeuroQuantology*, *20*(16), 5349–5359.

Jeon, Y., Jeon, H. S., Yi, C., Kwon, O., Cynn, H., & Oh, D. (2023). Effects of aquatic exercise on upper extremity function and postural control during reaching in children with cerebral palsy. *Physical Therapy Korea*, *30*(2), 128–135.

Kargarfard, M., Dehghadani, M., & Ghias, R. (2013). The effect of aquatic exercise therapy on muscle strength and joint's range of motion in hemophilia patients. *International Journal of Preventive Medicine*, *4*(1), 50–56.

Letieri, R. V., Furtado, G. E., Letieri, M., Góes, S. M., Pinheiro, C. J. B., Veronez, S. O., Magri, A. M., & Dantas, E. M. (2013). Pain, quality of life, self perception of health and depression in patients with fibromyalgia. *Revista Brasileira de Reumatologia*, *53*, 494–500.

Liu, Z., Huang, M., Liao, Y., Xie, X., Zhu, P., Liu, Y., & Tan, C. (2023). Long-term efficacy of hydrotherapy on balance function in patients with Parkinson's disease: A systematic review and meta-analysis. *Frontiers in Aging Neuroscience*, *15*, 1320240. https://doi.org/10.3389/fnagi.2023.1320240

Lawson, L. M., Foster, L., Harrington, M. C., & Oxley, C. A. (2014). Effects of a swim program for children with autism spectrum disorder on skills, interest, and participation in swimming. *American Journal of Recreation Therapy*, *13*(2), 17–27.

Ma, J., Zhang, T., He, Y., Li, X., Chen, H., & Zhao, Q. (2022). Effect of aquatic physical therapy on chronic low back pain: A systematic review and meta-analysis. *BMC Musculoskeletal Disorders*, *23*(1), 1050. https://doi.org/10.1186/s12891-022-05981-8

Marinho-Buzelli, A. R., Zaluski, A. J., Mansfield, A., Bonnyman, A. M., & Musselman, K. E. (2019). The use of aquatic therapy among rehabilitation professionals for individuals with spinal cord injury or disorder. *The Journal of Spinal Cord Medicine*, *42*(sup1), 158–165.

Mujawar, M. M. (2022). A systematic review of the effects of aquatic therapy on motor functions in children with cerebral palsy. *Reabilitacijos Mokslai: Slauga, Kineziterapija, Ergoterapija*, *2*(27), 51–67.

Muñoz-Blanco, E., Merino-Andrés, J., Aguilar-Soto, B., García, Y. C., Puente-Villalba, M., Pérez-Corrales, J., & Güeita-Rodríguez, J. (2020). Influence of aquatic therapy in children and youth with cerebral palsy: A qualitative case study in a special education school. *International Journal of Environmental Research and Public Health*, *17*(10), 3690.

Nissim, M., Ariel N., & Alter, E. (2022). Practical applications of aquatic physical activity, swimming, and therapy for people with visual impairment or blindness. *Movement*, *13*(3), 1–17.

Nissim, M., Rottenberg, Y., Karniel, N., & Ratzon, N. Z. (2024). Effects of aquatic exercise program versus on-land exercise program on cancer-related fatigue, neuropathy, activity and participation, quality of life, and return to work for cancer patients: Study protocol for a randomized controlled trial. *BMC Complementary Medicine and Therapies*, *24*(1), 74. https://doi.org/10.1186/s12906-024-04367-8

Oliver, M. (2018). A sociology of disability or a disablist sociology? In *Disability and Society* (pp. 18–42). Routledge.

Pérez-de la Cruz, S. (2019). Mental health in Parkinson's disease after receiving aquatic therapy: A clinical trial. *Acta Neurologica Belgica*, *119*, 193–200.

Pernambuco, C. S., Borba-Pinheiro, C. J., de Souza Vale, R. G., Di Masi, F., Monteiro, P. K. P., & Dantas, E. H. (2013). Functional autonomy, bone mineral density (BMD) and serum osteocalcin levels in older female participants of an aquatic exercise program (AAG). *Archives of Gerontology and Geriatrics*, *56*(3), 466–471.

Prabhu, C., & Dadmi, P. (2019). Effect of aquatic therapy v/s relaxation therapy in chronic low back pain. *International Journal of Orthopaedics Sciences*, *5*(1), 279–284.

Quraishi, S., & Jarrar, T. (2018). Impact of aquatic therapy on sensory modulation of autistic children to improve activities of daily living. *Pakistan Journal of Rehabilitation*, *7*(2), 13–18.

Rimmer, J. H., Riley, B., Wang, E., & Rauworth, A. (2005). Accessibility of health clubs for people with mobility disabilities and visual impairments. *American Journal of Public Health*, *95*(11), 2022–2028.

Sato, D., Yamashiro, K., Onishi, H., Shimoyama, Y., Yoshida, T., & Maruyama, A. (2012). The effect of water immersion on short-latency somatosensory evoked potentials in human. *BMC Neuroscience*, *13*, 1–6.

Shelef, A. N. (2010). Enhancing quality of life through aquatics therapy: Effectiveness of adaptation of seating posture loading in a partially immersed aquatics therapy approach for the improved functioning and perceived competence of children with cerebral palsy, as reflected in their quality of life: A multiple case study (Doctoral dissertation, Anglia Ruskin Research Online (ARRO)). Anglia Ruskin University.

Seligman, M. E., & Csikszentmihalyi, M. (2000). *Positive Psychology: An Introduction* (Vol. 55, No. 1, p. 5). American Psychological Association.

Stan, A. E. (2012). The benefits of participation in aquatic activities for people with disabilities. *Sports Medicine Journal/Medicina Sportivâ*, 8(1), 1737–1742.

Swain, J., & French, S. (2000). Towards an affirmation model of disability. *Disability & Society*, 15(4), 569–582.

Tufekcioglu, E., Arslan, D., Konukman, F., Zagorski, T., Al Batti, T., Filiz, B., … & Yilmaz, E. B. (2023). The Aquatic WATSU® Therapy Program Improves the Quality of Life of an Adult Male with Autism Spectrum Disorder. A Case Report. *Physical Culture and Sport*, 99(1), 11–20.

van Tulleken, C., Tipton, M., Massey, H., & Harper, C. M. (2018). Open water swimming as a treatment for major depressive disorder. *Case Reports*, 2018, bcr-2018. doi:10.1136/bcr-2018-225007.

Wilcock, I. M., Cronin, J. B., & Hing, W. A. (2006). Physiological response to water immersion: a method for sport recovery? *Sports Medicine*, 36, 747–765.

Xiang, A., Fu, Y., Wang, C., Huang, D., Qi, J., Zhao, R., Wu, L., Fan, C., & Zhang, Q. (2024). Aquatic therapy for spastic cerebral palsy: A scoping review. *European Journal of Medical Research*, 29(1), 569–575.

Zamunér, A. R., Andrade, C. P., Arca, E. A., & Avila, M. A. (2019). Impact of water therapy on pain management in patients with fibromyalgia: current perspectives. *Journal of Pain Research*, 12, 1971–2007. doi:https://org/10.2147/JPR.S161494

Chapter 5
Analysing Hydrotherapy Techniques Through the Lens of the Four-Dimensional Model

The Four-Dimensional Model of Hydrotherapy offers a comprehensive and structured framework for the analysis of hydrotherapy techniques. Grounded in an integrative view of rehabilitation, the model extends beyond biomechanical improvement to encompass psychological well-being, social participation and sustainable, person-centred outcomes. It emphasises the relational, emotional and social aspects of therapeutic practice, recognising rehabilitation as a multidimensional and transformative process. It invites practitioners to assess hydrotherapy methods through a lens that values not only physical gains, but also autonomy, emotional resilience, identity formation and long-term quality of life.

This chapter examines how a range of hydrotherapy techniques align with the model's four dimensions: (1) Body Functioning and Sensory Experience, (2) Affirmative Identity and Self-Determination, (3) Social Belonging and Inclusion, and (4) Holistic Well-Being and Long-Term Impact. Each dimension offers a distinct yet interconnected perspective for evaluating therapeutic interventions, ensuring that clinical practice remains holistic and responsive to participants' needs. Each technique is evaluated in terms of its capacity to support multidimensional therapeutic goals, including self-efficacy, functional autonomy and social connection.

The chapter highlights how the intentional application of this model can transform hydrotherapy from a set of clinical procedures into a meaningful, empowering and inclusive experience. By shifting from a deficit-oriented to an empowerment-oriented approach, practitioners can foster environments that nurture resilience, participation and personal agency. By adopting this holistic perspective, practitioners can optimise the therapeutic value of aquatic

DOI: 10.4324/9781003659709-8

interventions and ensure their relevance to the lived experiences and long-term aspirations of diverse participants.

WATSU

Body Functioning and Sensory Experience

Watsu (Water Shiatsu) aligns strongly with Dimension 1, as it utilises the physical properties of warm water (particularly buoyancy, hydrostatic pressure, and flowing, rhythmical movement) to facilitate mobility with minimal gravitational constraints. The technique reduces muscular tension, enhances joint range of motion, and supports proprioceptive integration, making it particularly beneficial for individuals with neurological impairments, sensory modulation difficulties, or chronic pain (Schitter et al., 2020). The continuous, three-dimensional movements provide consistent input to myofascial and vestibular systems, promoting postural alignment and neuromuscular relaxation. For individuals with heightened sensory defensiveness, Watsu has been shown to reduce discomfort and support sensory tolerance by delivering predictable and enveloping somatosensory input. The hydrostatic pressure of water also improves circulation and supports trunk stability, reinforcing Watsu's contribution to functional comfort and somatic awareness.

Affirmative Identity and Self-Determination

Watsu demonstrates moderate alignment with Dimension 2. While it is primarily a passive technique, its capacity to create a deeply supportive, non-judgmental environment allows individuals to experience their bodies in a positive and affirming way. By engaging in movement experiences that may otherwise be inaccessible on land, participants may develop increased self-awareness, comfort with bodily sensations, and confidence in their physical capabilities (Schitter et al., 2020). The predictability and rhythm of therapist-guided sequences can foster a sense of agency and trust, contributing to emotional regulation and resilience (Oh & Lee, 2011). In this way, Watsu supports psychological healing and identity formation, particularly among individuals living with trauma, anxiety, or chronic illness.

However, because Watsu does not require participants to initiate movement or set personal goals, it offers limited opportunities to develop functional autonomy or decision-making skills in therapy. While the technique fosters emotional empowerment and acceptance, its contribution to self-determined participation and skill-building is less robust than more active hydrotherapy modalities.

Social Belonging and Inclusion

Watsu does not inherently promote Dimension 3, as it is traditionally administered in one-on-one sessions and does not facilitate structured peer interaction. The absence of group-based components limits its ability to cultivate social belonging, teamwork, or shared therapeutic experiences. Nonetheless, Watsu may offer significant relational value through the therapeutic alliance it fosters. The technique relies on physical attunement, trust, and empathy between practitioner and participant, which may be particularly meaningful for individuals with histories of relational trauma or social isolation (Schitter et al., 2020). In community settings, Watsu could potentially be embedded into broader group programmes that include facilitated reflection or shared discussion, yet in its standard form, it offers only limited contributions to social inclusion.

Holistic Well-Being and Long-Term Impact

Watsu partially aligns with Dimension 4. Studies indicate that the technique supports autonomic nervous system regulation, reduces physiological markers of stress, and promotes improved sleep, emotional resilience, and mental well-being (Schitter et al., 2020; Oh & Lee, 2011). These outcomes may support participants in developing sustainable coping mechanisms for managing anxiety, pain, or fatigue. However, because Watsu is passive and practitioner-dependent, it does not equip individuals with transferable movement strategies, nor does it support long-term physical autonomy or independent engagement in exercise. Its long-term impact is therefore largely situated in the domains of psychological well-being and stress management, rather than in the cultivation of lifelong movement practices or functional independence.

AI CHI

Body Functioning and Sensory Experience

Ai Chi demonstrates strong alignment with Dimension 1, as it employs the physical properties of water (buoyancy, hydrostatic pressure, and resistance) to enhance postural control, proprioception, and motor coordination. Performed in shoulder-depth warm water, Ai Chi involves slow, continuous movements combined with diaphragmatic breathing. This setting facilitates improved joint mobility, muscle relaxation, and functional stability (Dunlap et al., 2021). Studies have shown that Ai Chi effectively reduces pain and improves balance in individuals with a range of neurological and musculoskeletal conditions, including Parkinson's disease, fibromyalgia, multiple sclerosis, and chronic back pain (Zamani & Rahnama, 2021; Pérez-de la Cruz et al., 2016).

The thermal and hydrostatic properties of the aquatic environment further support sensory integration, circulation, and pain modulation. Immersion to shoulder depth gently compresses the thorax, promoting respiratory expansion and endurance through diaphragmatic breathing (Becker, 2009). This breath-movement synchrony strengthens neuromuscular coordination and supports mind-body awareness, positioning Ai Chi as a holistic modality for sensory-motor rehabilitation.

Affirmative Identity and Self-Determination

Ai Chi moderately supports Dimension 2. Its flowing, mindful movements promote a sense of self-efficacy, body awareness, and emotional regulation. Participants are encouraged to move at their own pace, without judgement or external performance demands (Dunlap et al., 2021), fostering bodily acceptance and intrinsic motivation. The meditative aspects of Ai Chi, such as controlled breathing and focused attention, have been associated with reduced anxiety, improved sleep, and enhanced emotional resilience.

From a psychological perspective, Ai Chi aligns with principles of positive psychology and self-determination theory by providing empowering, affirming experiences. However, as a highly structured practice led by an instructor, it does not strongly emphasise autonomous movement planning or adaptive task modification. While participants develop confidence and inner calm, the opportunities for self-directed decision-making in movement are somewhat limited.

Social Belonging and Inclusion

Ai Chi aligns strongly with Dimension 3 through its inherently group-based format. The synchronised movement patterns, shared rhythms, and collective flow of participants contribute to a sense of interpersonal connection and non-verbal communication. As each participant's movement generates gentle ripples in the water, others subtly adjust, creating a dynamic of mutual responsiveness and shared experience.

This group synchrony fosters inclusion, empathy, and emotional attunement, particularly beneficial for individuals at risk of social withdrawal or isolation. The calm, non-competitive environment encourages equal participation, regardless of physical ability. Ai Chi thus creates a therapeutic space where participants feel seen, respected, and supported, reinforcing their sense of belonging within a group context.

Holistic Well-Being and Long-Term Impact

Ai Chi partially supports Dimension 4. It has been associated with sustained improvements in mental well-being, relaxation, and movement confidence (Dunlap et al., 2021). As a gentle, accessible practice, Ai Chi may be maintained over time as part of a wellness routine, promoting long-term engagement in health-promoting behaviours, particularly for individuals with chronic health conditions.

However, Ai Chi is not explicitly designed to facilitate the functional transfer of skills into everyday tasks. While it enhances self-awareness and promotes stress management, it does not directly target the development of task-specific functional independence or daily life participation. Its impact on long-term autonomy may therefore depend on how the practice is integrated into broader rehabilitation goals.

THE HALLIWICK CONCEPT

Body Functioning and Sensory Experience

The Halliwick Concept strongly aligns with Dimension 1, as it systematically integrates hydrostatics, hydrodynamics, and body mechanics to enhance motor control, balance, and postural stability (Garcia et al., 2012). The buoyant properties of water reduce gravitational load, enabling individuals with limited mobility to experience movement that may not be accessible on land. Hydrostatic pressure enhances proprioceptive input, supporting sensory awareness, postural alignment, and breath control.

A central component of the Halliwick Concept is its structured progression through water orientation, rotational control, and coordinated movement. This stepwise motor learning approach supports the development of independent movement, spatial awareness, and muscular control. Research has demonstrated particular benefits for children with cerebral palsy and individuals with neurological disabilities, including improved stability, voluntary movement initiation, and sensory-motor coordination (Kokaridas & Lambeck, 2015). Additionally, water resistance enables safe strength-building and tone regulation. Overall, Halliwick optimises postural control, sensory processing, and neuromuscular efficiency in water-based environments.

Affirmative Identity and Self-Determination

The Halliwick Concept strongly supports Dimension 2 by encouraging self-directed movement, autonomy, and gradual mastery. Through its ten-step programme, individuals progressively build movement confidence and a sense of control (Garcia et al., 2012). The absence of gravitational constraints creates a novel sense of freedom, often reducing anxiety and facilitating positive re-engagement with one's body.

Halliwick fosters experiences of physical competence and trust, aligning with the affirmative model of disability and self-determination theory (Bandura, 1997). Participants are supported to explore their capabilities rather than being defined by limitations, reinforcing emotional resilience and intrinsic motivation. The method's progressive reduction in therapist support encourages self-efficacy, enabling individuals to experience success through their own efforts. In doing so, Halliwick promotes a self-affirming identity grounded in autonomy and agency.

Social Belonging and Inclusion

The Halliwick Concept exhibits strong alignment with Dimension 3, as it is inherently group-based and rooted in inclusive practice. Sessions often bring together participants of different abilities, grouped by skill level rather than diagnosis, thereby reducing stigma and supporting social equality (Garcia et al., 2012). This reflects the social model of disability, which views exclusion as a result of structural and environmental barriers rather than individual impairments.

The aquatic environment further serves as a physical equaliser, as participants share a common horizontal level in water. This enhances peer interaction, mutual encouragement, and communication (Kokaridas & Lambeck, 2015). Structured group activities within Halliwick encourage cooperation, role-sharing, and positive interdependence. These elements support social confidence and provide a foundation for community participation beyond the therapeutic setting. As a practice often incorporated into adaptive swimming programmes, Halliwick supports both psychosocial well-being and broader inclusion.

Holistic Well-Being and Long-Term Impact

The Halliwick Concept demonstrates moderate alignment with Dimension 4. While its primary emphasis lies in motor learning and aquatic independence, it also contributes to sustained engagement in physical activity. Many individuals who gain confidence in Halliwick settings continue to participate in recreational swimming or community-based aquatic programmes, maintaining physical and emotional well-being over time.

Halliwick also contributes to long-term psychological outcomes, such as reduced anxiety and increased emotional resilience. From a lifespan perspective, the movement skills developed through Halliwick support fall prevention, functional posture, and participation in leisure activities. However, the technique does not directly target the transfer of aquatic skills to land-based functional mobility. As such, while it provides a strong foundation for lifelong engagement and empowerment, it may require complementary interventions to achieve broader daily life integration.

REHABILITATION SWIMMING: WATER WORLD SWIMMING THERAPY

Body Functioning and Sensory Experience

The Water World Swimming Therapy method demonstrates strong alignment with Dimension 1, as it enhances biomechanical efficiency while minimising physical strain. By individually tailoring swimming techniques to each person's unique anatomy and movement profile, Water World Swimming Therapy method reduces muscular tension, particularly in the neck and lower back, and promotes smooth, functional movement in water.

This person-centred approach leverages buoyancy and hydrostatic pressure to support postural alignment, joint unloading, and muscle relaxation. These properties are particularly valuable for individuals experiencing musculoskeletal and neurological conditions or chronic pain. The use of elongated strokes and slow, controlled breathing fosters proprioceptive input, flexibility, and endurance, reinforcing neuromuscular coordination and sensory integration.

The therapeutic benefits of warm water immersion further support circulation, reduce inflammation, and enhance overall movement quality. Together, these features position Water World Swimming Therapy method as a comprehensive therapeutic intervention that facilitates motor control and sensory-motor regulation in a low-impact, enriched environment.

Affirmative Identity and Self-Determination

The Water World Swimming Therapy aligns strongly with Dimension 2, as it shifts away from rigid, performance-driven swimming models in favour of individual adaptation. This approach emphasises the principle that movement should conform to the individual, not the reverse, creating space for self-directed learning, autonomy, and body trust.

Participants are encouraged to progress at their own pace, explore movement without pressure, and focus on comfort and confidence rather than external benchmarks. This adaptive philosophy fosters self-efficacy, resilience, and a positive relationship with the body. Rather than pathologising deviations from normative movement patterns, Water World Swimming Therapy method affirms diverse abilities and supports personal growth.

Although the method does not explicitly engage with disability identity discourse, it strongly reinforces agency, autonomy, and empowerment. By creating space for self-acceptance and adaptive success, Water World Swimming Therapy method aligns with affirmative and person-centred rehabilitation values.

Social Belonging and Inclusion

Water World Swimming Therapy method aligns strongly with Dimension 3, particularly through its emphasis on shared learning and group participation. Sessions are often delivered in inclusive settings that prioritise support, collaboration, and mutual encouragement over competition. This fosters a culture of belonging, where each individual is valued and progress is measured by personal growth rather than comparison.

The method's flexibility enables diverse participants to engage meaningfully, regardless of functional level, supporting the social model of disability. Rather than requiring conformity to a normative standard, Water World Swimming Therapy method adapts the swimming experience to fit the individual, removing structural barriers and reinforcing social participation.

Participants often report a strong sense of community, shared purpose, and reduced isolation. This peer-supported environment strengthens interpersonal bonds and contributes to emotional well-being, reinforcing the therapeutic and relational benefits of group-based aquatic activities.

Holistic Well-Being and Long-Term Impact

Water World Swimming Therapy method aligns strongly with Dimension 4, as it is explicitly designed for sustainability and lifelong engagement in physical activity. By equipping participants with adaptable swimming techniques, Water World Swimming Therapy method facilitates ongoing participation beyond formal therapy settings.

The method promotes injury prevention, emotional regulation, and physical confidence, making it suitable for individuals with chronic conditions or varying mobility levels. Participants often transition into recreational swimming, adaptive fitness programmes, or community-based aquatic activity, extending the benefits of hydrotherapy into everyday life.

Water World Swimming Therapy method's emphasis on self-paced, body-honouring movement enables individuals to develop routines that support long-term physical, emotional, and social well-being. In this way, Water World Swimming Therapy method serves not only as a rehabilitation tool but as a platform for empowerment, lifestyle adaptation, and health promotion across the lifespan.

THE BAD RAGAZ RING METHOD (BRRM)

Body Functioning and Sensory Experience

The Bad Ragaz Ring Method (BRRM) demonstrates strong alignment with Dimension 1, as it combines proprioceptive neuromuscular facilitation (PNF) principles with the unique therapeutic properties of water. Through the use of aquatic resistance, buoyancy, and viscosity, BRRM facilitates neuromuscular coordination, joint mobility, and progressive strength development (Rodica-Georgeta & Gheorghe, 2022).

Participants perform therapist-guided movements while supported by flotation devices (rings) around the neck, pelvis, or limbs. This setup allows for precise positioning and muscle activation while reducing gravitational load. Hydrostatic pressure enhances proprioceptive input, contributing to sensory integration, improved postural control, and circulation (Cha et al., 2017). BRRM is particularly effective for individuals with neurological conditions (e.g., stroke, spinal cord injury) and orthopaedic impairments, as it supports the re-education of functional movement patterns in a low-impact environment.

Affirmative Identity and Self-Determination

BRRM moderately aligns with Dimension 2. The method encourages skill acquisition and personal goal-setting through individually tailored resistance-based exercises. As participants gradually master complex movement patterns, they gain a sense of control, competence, and confidence in their physical abilities (Rodica-Georgeta & Gheorghe, 2022).

By fostering a sense of progress and achievement, BRRM reinforces self-efficacy and motivation, key elements in both self-determination theory and psychological resilience. However, the technique remains predominantly therapist-led, limiting opportunities for self-initiated exploration or autonomous movement planning. While BRRM supports empowerment through success in movement, it does not explicitly engage with identity-affirming practices or encourage expressive, participant-directed participation.

Social Belonging and Inclusion

BRRM shows limited alignment with Dimension 3, as it is typically delivered in an individualised, one-on-one format. While this format facilitates a strong therapeutic alliance, characterised by trust, emotional safety, and attunement between therapist and participant, it does not inherently support peer interaction, group collaboration, or shared experiences (Garcia et al., 2012).

For individuals who benefit from close professional guidance, BRRM offers a safe and responsive environment. However, from a social inclusion perspective, the absence of structured group engagement and collective participation limits the method's potential to foster social belonging, teamwork, or broader community integration.

Holistic Well-Being and Long-Term Impact

BRRM aligns moderately with Dimension 4, particularly through its focus on neuromuscular re-education, balance training, and injury prevention. The method supports functional independence in land-based tasks such as gait, standing balance, and reaching. Moreover, BRRM can reduce the risk of secondary complications, including muscle atrophy, joint contractures, and postural asymmetries, that often accompany chronic conditions (Rodica-Georgeta & Gheorghe, 2022).

Participants frequently report psychological benefits such as pain relief, enhanced mood, and improved movement confidence (So et al., 2019). These factors contribute to a more positive relationship with physical activity and a willingness to remain engaged in rehabilitation. Nonetheless, since BRRM is therapist-guided and relies on external facilitation, its impact on long-term autonomous participation and independent exercise may be limited unless followed by self-directed programmes or community-based adaptations.

AQUA STRETCH

Body Functioning and Sensory Experience

Aqua Stretch aligns strongly with Dimension 1 as it targets fascial adhesions and soft tissue restrictions through guided stretching techniques performed in a supportive aquatic environment. The method combines elements of assisted stretching, myofascial release, and therapist-guided resistance with the properties of water (buoyancy, viscosity, and hydrostatic pressure) to facilitate greater range of motion, pain reduction, and neuromuscular re-education (Kochar, 2011).

The aquatic setting allows for deeper and more sustained flexibility gains than land-based stretching due to the reduction of gravitational load. Participants experience enhanced circulation, muscle relaxation, and reduced soft tissue tension, making Aqua Stretch particularly beneficial for individuals recovering from orthopaedic surgery or managing chronic musculoskeletal pain (Pandya et al., 2021). Additionally, the continuous proprioceptive input provided by hydrostatic pressure and movement in water enhances body awareness and functional mobility.

Affirmative Identity and Self-Determination

Aqua Stretch demonstrates moderate alignment with Dimension 2. Unlike fully passive stretching modalities, Aqua Stretch encourages participants to actively guide and modulate their movement responses, fostering a sense of autonomy and self-regulation (Soufivand et al., 2024). The collaborative nature of the technique enables individuals to communicate their comfort levels, adjust intensity, and explore movement within a safe and responsive environment.

By reducing fear of movement and pain, Aqua Stretch helps restore trust in one's body and builds perceived self-efficacy, especially among individuals with long-standing mobility limitations. However, while the method promotes control and progress in movement, it does not explicitly engage with broader psychological constructs such as identity affirmation, emotional resilience, or self-expression, elements central to the affirmative disability model. As such, its contribution to identity development is supportive but limited in scope.

Social Belonging and Inclusion

Aqua Stretch demonstrates limited alignment with Dimension 3, as it is typically delivered in a one-on-one therapeutic format. This individualised approach facilitates focused and adaptive support, allowing for trust and emotional safety within the therapist–participant relationship. However, Aqua Stretch does not inherently incorporate peer interaction, group collaboration, or communal experiences, which are essential components of social belonging.

Although the intervention may indirectly contribute to emotional connection through the therapeutic alliance, it does not provide a structured setting for peer engagement or social inclusion. For individuals who require or prefer personalised intervention, Aqua Stretch offers a meaningful experience of support and attunement, but its capacity to foster group-based inclusion or shared belonging remains limited.

Holistic Well-Being and Long-Term Impact

Aqua Stretch aligns moderately with Dimension 4. Research suggests that regular participation in Aqua Stretch may yield sustained improvements in pain management, functional mobility, and sleep quality, as well as reductions in fatigue (Soufivand et al., 2024). By releasing fascial restrictions and improving movement efficiency, the method contributes to long-term musculoskeletal health and supports the prevention of secondary complications, such as joint stiffness or postural imbalances.

Nonetheless, Aqua Stretch is primarily a therapist-facilitated intervention rather than a self-directed practice. It does not inherently provide participants with tools for ongoing independent movement or a structured programme for long-term engagement beyond the clinical setting. While it may serve as an effective adjunct within a broader rehabilitation or wellness plan, its sustainability depends on continued access to therapist-led sessions or integration with more autonomous aquatic activities.

DEEP-WATER RUNNING

Body Functioning and Sensory Experience

Deep-water running (DWR) aligns strongly with Dimension 1, offering a low-impact cardiovascular workout within a buoyant, non-weight-bearing aquatic environment. The buoyancy of water significantly reduces ground reaction forces and minimises joint loading, making it particularly beneficial for individuals experiencing joint pain, recovering from injury, or facing mobility challenges (Kwok et al., 2022).

The properties of water, including hydrostatic pressure and multidirectional resistance, create an environment that challenges postural stability and requires engagement of multiple muscle groups (Meredith-Jones et al., 2009), these conditions are likely to activate deep stabilising muscles and support neuromuscular coordination during movement. Research indicates that DWR can effectively improve cardiorespiratory fitness and functional mobility, particularly in older adults, sedentary individuals, and athletes. Evidence suggests improvements in walking performance (Kwok et al., 2022).

Affirmative Identity and Self-Determination

Deep-Water Running demonstrates moderate alignment with Dimension 2. By enabling individuals to engage in physically demanding exercise without joint strain, DWR supports a sense of competence, agency, and safe physical challenge. Deep-water running is particularly suitable for individuals recovering from injury or managing chronic pain, as it enables participation in aerobic activity without placing excessive load on joints or exacerbating symptoms. This may support continued engagement in physical fitness and promote positive experiences in movement (Kwok et al., 2022; Meredith-Jones et al., 2009).

The adaptability of DWR supports progressive, self-paced goal-setting, reinforcing self-efficacy and encouraging long-term exercise engagement. Participants are able to regain or maintain an active lifestyle, which contributes to personal resilience and a positive relationship with one's body. However, while the method fosters confidence and functional autonomy, it does not directly engage with emotional identity, self-concept, or disability affirmation, key components of this dimension. Thus, DWR supports functional self-determination more than it advances identity formation or expressive empowerment.

Social Belonging and Inclusion

Deep-Water Running aligns strongly with Dimension 3, when practiced in group settings. Group-based DWR promotes shared rhythm, motivation, and peer interaction, which are key to building emotional support and community connection.

The inclusive nature of DWR enables individuals with diverse physical abilities and fitness levels to participate equitably. The aquatic setting minimises visual and functional differences between participants, reducing barriers related to appearance, movement style, or endurance. This encourages participation among individuals who may feel excluded from land-based fitness environments. Moreover, DWR groups promote accountability, mutual encouragement, and a sense of shared progress, key facilitators of social inclusion and psychological safety.

Holistic Well-Being and Long-Term Impact

DWR demonstrates strong alignment with Dimension 4, serving as a sustainable form of cardiovascular and muscular training that can be continued well beyond rehabilitation. aerobic fitness and functional mobility, particularly in older and sedentary adults, with potential benefits for maintaining independence in daily activities (Kwok et al., 2022).

In addition to its physical benefits, DWR supports emotional regulation, stress reduction, and improved well-being. One study reported enhanced mental health scores following a DWR intervention (Kwok et al., 2022). Notably, DWR is a self-directed and scalable intervention that does not require continuous therapist involvement, increasing its potential for integration into regular health routines. As such, it supports lifelong physical activity, emotional wellness, and community participation, hallmarks of holistic rehabilitation.

INTEGRATING THE FOUR-DIMENSIONAL MODEL ACROSS HYDROTHERAPY TECHNIQUES: A REFLECTIVE SUMMARY

By applying the Four-Dimensional Model of Hydrotherapy, each technique presented in this chapter has been evaluated not only for its contribution to Body Functioning and Sensory Experience but also for its role in promoting Affirmative Identity and Self-Determination, Social Belonging and Inclusion, and Holistic Well-Being and Long-Term Impact. This structured yet flexible framework highlights the diverse therapeutic potentials of hydrotherapy, revealing how different techniques prioritise various dimensions according to their underlying philosophy and clinical application.

Importantly, the model distinguishes between intentional impacts and incidental or secondary outcomes. For example, a method that primarily supports physical functioning may also, as a secondary effect, improve psychological well-being or foster inclusion, even if these effects are not explicitly cultivated by the therapist. Conversely, when certain dimensions are overlooked or remain unacknowledged, they may not only fail to develop but may also become unintentionally constrained. For instance, techniques that promote physical dependency without addressing autonomy and agency may inadvertently inhibit self-determination or reinforce passive therapeutic roles.

Because the four dimensions are conceptualised as interwoven and dynamic rather than as linear stages, targeted progress in one area may catalyse growth across others. However, without a conscious, person-centred approach, these interdimensional influences may remain underutilised or inconsistently aligned. The model thus serves not only as an analytical lens but also as a reflective tool, encouraging practitioners to identify potential blind spots, clarify their therapeutic intentions, and intentionally broaden the scope of their interventions.

This comparative framework enables hydrotherapists and interdisciplinary teams to critically evaluate each technique's alignment with broader psychosocial, emotional, and rehabilitative goals. In doing so, it ensures that intervention planning remains inclusive, intentional, and responsive to the diverse needs, aspirations, and identities of individuals. A visual summary of the techniques' relative alignment with the Four-Dimensional Model is presented in Table 5.1.

Table 5.1 Analysing Hydrotherapy Techniques Through the Lens of the Four-Dimensional Model

Hydrotherapy Technique	Body Functioning and Sensory Experience	Affirmative Identity and Self-Determination	Social Belonging and Inclusion	Holistic Well-Being and Long-Term Impact
Halliwick Concept	Strong	Strong	Strong	Moderate
Bad Ragaz Ring Method	Strong	Moderate	Limited	Moderate
Ai Chi	Strong	Moderate	Strong	Partial
Deep-Water Running	Strong	Moderate	Strong	Strong
Rehabilitation Swimming: Water World Swimming Therapy	Strong	Strong	Strong	Strong
Watsu	Strong	Moderate	Limited	Partial
AquaStretch	Strong	Moderate	Limited	Moderate

Ultimately, the integration of the Four-Dimensional Model into hydrotherapy practice enhances both clinical effectiveness and humanistic care. It reframes hydrotherapy not solely as a modality for physical rehabilitation but as a transformative space for empowerment, emotional flourishing, social connection, and sustained participation across the lifespan.

REFERENCES

Bandura, A. (1997). *Self-efficacy: The Exercise of Control*. Freeman.

Becker, B. E. (2009). Aquatic therapy: Scientific foundations and clinical rehabilitation applications. *PM&R, 1*(9), 859–872.

Cha, H. G., Kim, M. K., & Jung, J. H. (2017). Effects of Bad Ragaz Ring method on balance and walking ability in patients with post-stroke hemiparesis. *Journal of Physical Therapy Science, 29*(2), 313–317.

Dunlap, E., Lambeck, J., Ku, P. H., & Gobert, D. (2021). Ai Chi for balance, pain, functional mobility, and quality of life in adults: a scoping review. *The Journal of Aquatic Physical Therapy, 29*(1), 14–28.

Garcia, J. M., da Silva, L. S., & Alves, A. L. (2012). The Halliwick Concept: Swimming instruction and therapy for individuals with disabilities. *Brazilian Journal of Physical Therapy*, *16*(2), 108–115.

Kochar, R. D. (2011). Effect of AquaStretch on range of motion at knee joint in total knee arthroplasty patients. *Journal of Musculoskeletal Research*, *14*(2), 145–156.

Kokaridas, D., & Lambeck, J. (2015). The effectiveness of the Halliwick Concept in aquatic therapy for children with cerebral palsy. *European Journal of Adapted Physical Activity*, *8*(1), 20–35.

Kwok, M. M., So, B. C., Heywood, S., Lai, M. C., & Ng, S. S. (2022). Effectiveness of deep water running on improving cardiorespiratory fitness, physical function and quality of life: A systematic review. *International Journal of Environmental Research and Public Health*, *19*(15), 9434.

Meredith-Jones, K., Legge, M., & Jones, L. M. (2009). Circuit-based deep water running improves cardiovascular fitness, strength and abdominal obesity in older, overweight women. *Med Sport*, *13*(1), 5–12.

Oh, J. S., & Lee, S. K. (2011). Stress relieving effects of Watsu. *Kor J Aesthet Cosmetol*, *9*(3), 1–9.

Pandya, E., Makhecha, K., & Patel, A. (2021). Comparing short term effect of aqua stretch with supervised land-based stretching in chronic non-specific neck pain among young working female physiotherapists: A randomized clinical trial. *International Journal of Current Research and Review*, *13*(12), 160–167.

Pérez-De La Cruz, S., Luengo, A. G., & Lambeck, J. (2016). Effects of an Ai Chi fall prevention programme for patients with Parkinson's disease. *Neurología* (English Edition), *31*(3), 176–182.

Rodica-Georgeta, C., & Gheorghe, P. (2022). The effectiveness of the Bad Ragaz Ring Method in neuromuscular rehabilitation: A systematic review. *European Journal of Physical Therapy*, *28*(4), 512–526.

Schitter, A. M., Fleckenstein, J., Frei, P., Taeymans, J., Kurpiers, N., & Radlinger, L. (2020). Applications, indications, and effects of passive hydrotherapy WATSU (WaterShiatsu): A systematic review and meta-analysis. *PLoS One*, *15*(3), e0229705.

So, B. C., Kwok, M. L., & Fong, K. (2019). The effects of Bad Ragaz Ring Method on balance and mobility in stroke survivors. *International Journal of Physical Medicine & Rehabilitation*, *7*(4), 356–368.

Soufivand, P., Gandomi, F., Assar, S., Abbasi, H., Salimi, M., Ezati, M., & Shahsavari, S. (2024). The effect of a six-week Aqua Pilates and Aqua Stretch intervention on pain, function, and quality of life in patients affected by ankylosing spondylitis: A rater-blind randomized controlled trial. *Journal of Back and Musculoskeletal Rehabilitation*, *37*(1), 1–12.

Zamani, J., & Rahnama, N. (2021). The effect of Ai Chi and Tai Chi training on physical function, functional balance and fear of falling of patients with knee osteoarthritis. *Feyz, Journal of Kashan University of Medical Sciences*, *24*(6), 611–620.

Part III

Practice

Case Reports and Future Directions

Chapter 6
Case Reports Using the Four-Dimensional Model

Case reports serve as a crucial and nuanced tool for documenting individualised and context-sensitive rehabilitation processes. They offer rich insight into how therapeutic strategies are applied and experienced in diverse, real-world settings (Gagnier et al., 2013). Within the field of hydrotherapy, such reports support evidence-informed clinical reflection, allow for the refinement of therapeutic practices, and contribute to evaluating outcomes that are not only functionally meaningful but also aligned with the individual's own values and lived experiences.

The present chapter introduces a series of case reports analysed through the Four-Dimensional Model of Hydrotherapy – a holistic and person-centred framework designed to assess rehabilitation beyond conventional biomechanical recovery. This model allows for a layered interpretation of change, recognising that physical, emotional, social, and long-term outcomes are interdependent and dynamic.

The CARE (CAse REport) guidelines (Riley et al., 2017) provide the foundation for structuring these reports, ensuring methodological transparency, ethical clarity, and reporting consistency. Each case follows a standardised format, incorporating a contextual history of the individual, relevant functional and psychosocial assessments, the therapeutic approach, and follow-up outcomes. By adhering to internationally recognised reporting standards, this chapter contributes to the growing literature on hydrotherapy's role in rehabilitation, while reinforcing the integration of lived experience into clinical reasoning.

Each report is systematically analysed through the lens of the Four-Dimensional Model of Hydrotherapy, which offers a structured yet adaptable framework for understanding progress across physical, emotional, social, and long-term domains:

DOI: 10.4324/9781003659709-10

- Body Functioning and Sensory Experience: Considers the effects of hydrotherapy on musculoskeletal function, proprioception, postural control, and sensory integration. It highlights the contribution of the aquatic environment in supporting safe, adaptive, and confident movement.
- Affirmative Identity and Self-Determination: Explores how therapeutic experiences influence self-efficacy, autonomy, emotional regulation, and the development of a positive, empowered disability identity.
- Social Belonging and Inclusion: Assesses the ways in which hydrotherapy fosters social interaction, emotional well-being, and a sense of shared experience, either in group-based contexts or through relational processes with practitioners.
- Holistic Well-Being and Long-Term Impact: Evaluates the sustainability and broader life relevance of outcomes, including maintenance of functional gains, participation in meaningful activities, and long-term strategies for health, inclusion, and personal growth.

By applying this multidimensional framework, the case reports in this chapter move beyond symptom management or isolated functional gains. They offer insight into the lived rehabilitation journey, including processes of identity formation, self-advocacy, and participation. In doing so, they position hydrotherapy not only as a clinical intervention but as a means of facilitating autonomy, resilience, and community integration. The reflections derived from these narratives are intended to support evidence-informed practice and guide clinicians, researchers, and educators in embedding hydrotherapy within inclusive, holistic models of care.

APPLYING THE FOUR-DIMENSIONAL MODEL OF HYDROTHERAPY IN THE REHABILITATION OF A 25-YEAR-OLD MAN FOLLOWING A KNEE LIGAMENT INJURY

Abstract

Background: Knee ligament injuries, particularly anterior cruciate ligament (ACL) ruptures, pose complex rehabilitation challenges due to biomechanical instability and psychosocial disruption. Hydrotherapy is increasingly recognised as a multidimensional intervention supporting both functional and emotional recovery.

Case Presentation: This report describes the rehabilitation of a 25-year-old man who sustained an ACL rupture, medial meniscal tear, and chondral damage following a road traffic accident. Post-surgical rehabilitation incorporated a structured 12-week hydrotherapy programme, evaluated using the Four-Dimensional Model of Hydrotherapy.

Intervention: The hydrotherapy intervention focused on restoring mobility, neuromuscular control, proprioception, and psychological resilience. The programme progressed from buoyancy-assisted gait training and proprioceptive drills to group-based dynamic activities and deep-water plyometric exercises.

Outcomes: The individual exhibited notable improvements in joint function, strength symmetry (LSI improved from 60% to 74%), pain reduction (VAS decreased from 7/10 to 3/10), and decreased fear of movement (TSK-11 score reduced from 35 to 25). Psychosocially, a shift was observed from a highly centralised athletic identity to a more adaptive and integrated self-concept.

Conclusion: Hydrotherapy supported recovery across physical, emotional, and identity domains. The Four-Dimensional Model provided a person-centred framework for evaluating whole-person outcomes in rehabilitation.

Keywords: ACL injury; athletic identity; case report; hydrotherapy; psychological adaptation; rehabilitation

Introduction

Musculoskeletal conditions involving the knee are among the most frequently encountered challenges in physical rehabilitation. Injuries such as anterior cruciate ligament (ACL) ruptures and meniscal tears affect individuals across a wide range of activity levels (Amras & Kamalakannan, 2023). Given the biomechanical complexity of the knee and its central role in movement and weight-bearing, recovery often requires personalised, interdisciplinary approaches (Zhang et al., 2020).

Hydrotherapy has emerged as a valuable component of rehabilitation following knee injury, offering a supportive sensory-motor environment that facilitates early mobilisation while reducing physical strain. Buoyancy allows for movement with minimal joint compression, hydrostatic pressure supports proprioceptive feedback and oedema management, and the warm aquatic environment contributes to pain relief and muscle relaxation (Buckthorpe et al., 2019; Hajouj et al., 2021). Evidence suggests that incorporating water-based therapy into recovery programmes can enhance functional mobility, reduce pain, and improve neuromuscular coordination following ACL reconstruction or meniscal repair (Amras & Kamalakannan, 2023; McAvoy, 2009).

This case report describes the hydrotherapy journey of a 25-year-old man recovering from a knee ligament injury, focusing on the use of a structured aquatic intervention to support his physical, emotional, and functional progress. His rehabilitation is analysed using the Four-Dimensional Model of Hydrotherapy, which provides a holistic framework for assessing outcomes across:

1. Body Functioning and Sensory Experience - examining the impact of hydrotherapy on musculoskeletal recovery, proprioception, and sensory regulation.
2. Affirmative Identity and Self-Determination - exploring how engaging in movement and goal-directed therapy supports self-confidence, autonomy, and positive identity development.
3. Social Belonging and Inclusion - assessing the role of hydrotherapy in fostering emotional well-being, interpersonal connection, and shared therapeutic experience.
4. Holistic Well-Being and Long-Term Impact - evaluating how the gains made in hydrotherapy translate to everyday life, sustainable activity, and long-term quality of life.

By applying this multidimensional lens, the case illustrates how water-based rehabilitation can serve not only as a tool for physical recovery, but also as a means for emotional empowerment, identity reinforcement, and inclusive, person-centred care.

Participant Information[1]

The individual, a 25-year-old who had been actively engaged in competitive soccer and high-intensity training, initiated rehabilitation following a right knee injury sustained in a high-impact road accident. Prior to the injury, his daily routine and personal identity were closely tied to physical activity and athletic performance.

The accident resulted in a complex knee injury, including a complete ACL rupture, medial meniscus tear, and cartilage damage to the femoral condyle. These injuries necessitated surgical intervention. The individual underwent arthroscopic ACL reconstruction using a hamstring tendon autograft, along with partial medial meniscectomy and chondroplasty.

Beyond its physical consequences, the injury had notable psychosocial and identity-related implications. The individual previously identified strongly with his athletic role, and the injury disrupted both his functional independence and his sense of self. Following surgery, he expressed uncertainty regarding his ability to return to competitive sports and concern about the future of his athletic involvement. His baseline score on the Tampa Scale of Kinesiophobia (TSK-11) was 35, reflecting a high level of fear-avoidance beliefs (Woby et al., 2005).

The transition from full independence to temporarily requiring mobility assistance and support with daily activities affected not only his functional capacity but also his emotional resilience. He reported experiencing reduced confidence, apprehension regarding sudden movements, and anxiety about potential graft failure. During the initial post-surgical evaluation, he demonstrated difficulty in weight-bearing tasks such as walking, stair climbing, and maintaining dynamic knee stability, all of which impacted his perceived autonomy and body trust.

Health and Functional Profile[2]

A comprehensive physical assessment was conducted to evaluate joint integrity, movement quality, and pain response in the affected knee. Marked joint effusion and swelling were observed, contributing to restricted active and passive range of motion. At the start of rehabilitation, knee flexion was limited to 90° and extension to −5°, with discomfort reported during both movements. The Lachman and anterior drawer tests were positive, consistent with anterior cruciate ligament (ACL) insufficiency (Sokal et al., 2022). Medial joint line tenderness suggested meniscal involvement, while valgus stress testing indicated possible medial ligament instability.

The individual rated his pain as 7 out of 10 on the Visual Analogue Scale (VAS), particularly during weight-bearing tasks. Isokinetic dynamometry revealed a significant quadriceps strength deficit, with the injured limb demonstrating approximately 50% of the strength of the non-injured side. The Limb Symmetry Index (LSI) was 60%, indicating reduced neuromuscular coordination and asymmetry. Functional assessments, such as the single-leg hop test, confirmed impaired explosive strength and landing stability.

In addition to these physical findings, the individual expressed psychological distress related to his sudden loss of athletic function. Having previously identified strongly with a competitive football role, he reported a sense of disconnection from his athletic identity. His score on the Athletic Identity Measurement Scale (AIMS) was 50 out of 70, reflecting a deeply internalised athletic identity characterised by emotional investment in sport and a sense of belonging to the athletic community. While this identity remained present, the injury had introduced doubt, emotional strain, and a decline in movement confidence.

Imaging studies confirmed the clinical picture. Magnetic Resonance Imaging (MRI) showed a complete ACL rupture, medial meniscus tear, and chondral damage to the femoral condyle. No bony fractures were detected. Post-traumatic synovitis was noted, contributing to persistent joint swelling and discomfort.

Given the extent of structural damage and its impact on mobility and participation, arthroscopic ACL reconstruction was performed using a hamstring tendon autograft- a procedure widely recommended for young, physically active individuals. A partial medial meniscectomy was undertaken to remove unstable tissue, and focal chondroplasty addressed cartilage damage.

Following surgery, the individual was fitted with a hinged knee brace, initially limiting flexion to 90° and extension to 0°, to protect the graft during early healing. A progressive weight-bearing protocol was introduced, beginning with 10 days of non-weight-bearing mobilisation and advancing to partial loading. Early physiotherapy targeted oedema control, pain reduction, and quadriceps activation. A structured range-of-motion programme was initiated alongside neuromuscular retraining to reduce asymmetry and restore functional movement.

Therapeutic Intervention

Following arthroscopic ACL reconstruction with a hamstring tendon autograft, partial medial meniscectomy, and chondroplasty, the individual commenced a land-based physiotherapy programme aimed at early-stage recovery. During the initial four to six weeks post-surgery, rehabilitation focused on managing oedema, activating the quadriceps, and gradually introducing weight-bearing exercises within a structured and supportive framework.

While incremental improvements in mobility were noted, challenges remained- particularly persistent knee stiffness, heightened anxiety during load-bearing tasks, and psychological unease surrounding high-impact movement. These difficulties reflected not only physical limitations but also a reduced sense of body confidence and fear of reinjury.

To address these interconnected needs, a structured hydrotherapy programme was introduced as a complementary phase in the individual's rehabilitation. The aquatic environment was selected to reduce joint loading, support safe movement exploration, and foster emotional regulation -creating space for progress both physically and psychologically.

The hydrotherapy programme was implemented as a 12-week structured intervention, divided into three progressive phases. Each phase was designed to support gradual, safe reintegration into functional movement, with a focus on enhancing joint stability, neuromuscular control, proprioceptive awareness, and emotional confidence. The progression was carefully paced to reflect the individual's evolving capabilities and comfort, balancing physical challenge with psychological readiness.

Early Recovery Phase (Weeks 7–10 Post-Surgery)

During this phase, the primary aim was to alleviate postoperative stiffness, improve joint mobility, and re-establish proprioceptive awareness within a safe and supported environment. The properties of water – particularly buoyancy and hydrostatic pressure – were utilised to facilitate movement with reduced pain and minimal strain on healing tissues. Buoyancy-assisted knee mobilisation enabled passive and assisted flexion and extension exercises, reducing gravitational loading and supporting controlled motion without overloading the ACL graft.

Gait retraining in water provided the opportunity for progressive weight-bearing, while maintaining joint alignment and dynamic stability. Hydrostatic pressure further promoted circulation, reduced oedema, and alleviated stiffness, while the warm-water environment contributed to muscle relaxation and overall ease of movement.

Proprioceptive and balance drills, enhanced by gentle water turbulence, were introduced to activate joint-stabilising responses and deepen sensory awareness. Given the individual's psychological hesitancy and fear of re-injury, gradual exposure strategies – such as reintroducing previously avoided movements like walking or jumping in a gravity-reduced setting – were employed alongside breath control techniques to reduce anxiety and restore a sense of bodily trust. These components not only supported physical adaptation but also strengthened self-efficacy and emotional readiness for continued participation in the recovery journey.

Intermediate Recovery Phase (Weeks 11–14 Post-Surgery)

During this phase, rehabilitation focused on strength development, functional stability, and the reintroduction of controlled impact. Resistance-based strength training utilised the viscosity of water to progressively engage the quadriceps, hamstrings, and core stabilisers. With increasing mobility, water jets and aquatic equipment- including pool noodles, fins, and ankle weights-were incorporated to enhance targeted muscular activation.

Proprioceptive neuromuscular facilitation included single-leg balance exercises, perturbation drills, and coordinated movement sequences aimed at enhancing neuromuscular control. Deep-water walking and running simulations with flotation belts offered high-intensity, low-impact cardiovascular conditioning while supporting postural alignment and trunk control.

Functional closed-chain movements, such as partial squats, step-ups, and controlled lunges, were adapted to the aquatic environment to maximise muscle engagement with minimal joint compression. Sport-specific retraining was gradually introduced, with water-based exercises simulating soccer-related movement patterns. These drills supported a safe return to dynamic loading and directional control, reinforcing physical confidence and readiness for more advanced tasks.

Late Recovery Phase (Weeks 15–18 Post-Surgery)

The final phase focused on the transition from controlled aquatic therapy to full weight-bearing, land-based rehabilitation, supporting a safe return to recreational and sport-specific activities. Deep-water training, including explosive jumps, acceleration drills, and controlled landings, was employed to enhance neuromuscular coordination and force absorption while minimising joint strain.

Agility-focused drills incorporated lateral movements, rapid directional changes, and multidirectional challenges to restore reaction time, dynamic balance, and joint control. To enhance motivation and adaptability, group-based exercises were introduced into the hydrotherapy programme. Paired tasks, such as buoyant ball passing during jump sequences, supported neuromuscular timing and movement precision. Mirror agility drills, wherein one participant mimicked the movements of another, further developed proprioceptive awareness and reaction capabilities.

Dynamic resistance challenges using aquatic bands in small groups targeted core engagement and lower-limb control under varying force directions. These paired activities directly supported the subdimension of group cooperation (3b), fostering movement confidence through socially meaningful and cooperative aquatic interaction. The group setting contributed to a sense of belonging and emotional support, reinforcing motivation and reducing the emotional burden of recovery.

To facilitate a smooth transition to land-based therapy, hydrotherapy sessions were integrated with traditional physiotherapy through a gradual reduction in immersion depth. This strategic approach systematically increased gravitational load, enhancing musculoskeletal readiness and neuromotor adaptation. The stepwise return, from deep to shallow water and then to dry land, enabled the individual to rebuild strength, joint stability, and movement confidence while reducing the risk of re-injury and fear avoidance.

Follow-up and Outcomes

At the 12-week follow-up, the individual demonstrated measurable improvements in knee function, although deficits in strength, dynamic stability, and psychological readiness for high-impact activities remained.

An isokinetic dynamometry test was conducted to assess quadriceps and hamstring strength in both legs. The results indicated that the injured leg had regained approximately 75% of the strength of the non-injured limb, compared to pre-hydrotherapy levels of 50%. While this represented substantial progress, it remained below the recommended 90% threshold for safe return to high-demand sports. The hamstring-to-quadriceps (H/Q) ratio of the injured limb was 0.54, improving from the pre-rehabilitation score of 0.48 but still not reaching the optimal 0.6–0.7 ratio associated with dynamic knee stability.

A single-leg hop test was used to evaluate functional symmetry. The individual achieved a Limb Symmetry Index (LSI) of 74%, a marked improvement from the initial 60%, indicating better neuromuscular control. Hop test distance on the injured limb reached 80% of the non-injured side, up from 60% pre-rehabilitation, demonstrating increased explosive strength and landing control.

Pain levels decreased, with Visual Analog Scale (VAS) scores dropping from 7/10 at the start of hydrotherapy to 3/10 by week 12. Passive range of motion assessments showed near-full restoration of knee flexion (125°) and extension (-2°), although mild stiffness persisted after prolonged activity. Joint effusion significantly decreased, with no clinical signs of synovitis. Mild residual swelling was observed following extended weight-bearing tasks but did not interfere with functional movement.

Repeat Lachman and valgus stress tests showed significant improvements in knee stability. The Lachman test demonstrated a firm endpoint with minimal anterior translation, suggesting restored ACL integrity. The valgus stress test was negative for medial instability, indicating effective rehabilitation of ligamentous structures.

Despite these physical gains, the individual reported lingering psychological apprehension about returning to high-impact or competitive activity. His Tampa Scale of Kinesiophobia (TSK-11) score declined from 35 to 25, suggesting reduced fear of movement, but he continued to hesitate with unilateral loading and sport-specific drills.

From a psychosocial perspective, a notable shift occurred in the individual's athletic identity. His post-intervention score on the Athletic Identity Measurement Scale (AIMS) was estimated at 41 out of 70, down from a pre-intervention score of 50. This reflects a moderated but still present athletic self-concept, with a gradual transition from an exclusive athletic identity toward a more balanced sense of self. The individual continued to view himself as a physically active person but was beginning to explore alternative ways to express and experience this identity. This evolving perspective on physical identity reflects a shift toward long-term adaptation and well-being, as the individual began to reframe his athleticism within a broader, sustainable life context.

Although he successfully reintegrated into daily routines and light recreational sport, a full return to competitive soccer was not recommended at this stage due to persisting asymmetries, incomplete strength restoration. He was advised to continue progressive strength training and neuromuscular re-education to optimise long-term outcomes and reduce the risk of reinjury.

Discussion

The rehabilitation of ACL injuries and meniscal tears is a complex and multidimensional journey that extends beyond biomechanical recovery alone. While land-based physiotherapy is widely regarded as a cornerstone of post-surgical recovery following ACL reconstruction (Rosenblatt et al., 2008; Zaffagnini et al., 2015), hydrotherapy offers a valuable and person-centred complement. By harnessing the physical and sensory properties of water, hydrotherapy supports early mobilisation, neuromuscular re-education, emotional regulation, and progressive re-engagement with movement, all within a low-impact and psychologically supportive environment.

This case report explored the outcomes of a structured 12-week aquatic intervention using the Four-Dimensional Model of Hydrotherapy, offering a holistic lens through which to understand physical, emotional, social, and long-term recovery processes.

Body Functioning and Sensory Experience

The individual demonstrated clear gains in muscular strength, proprioceptive awareness, range of motion, and pain reduction. Hydrostatic pressure contributed significantly to controlling oedema and enhancing circulation, while buoyancy enabled early mobilisation without overloading healing tissues. Nonetheless, the individual had not yet reached the commonly recommended 90% functional symmetry threshold for return to high-impact sport. Although the hamstring-to-quadriceps (H/Q) ratio improved from 0.48 to 0.54, further neuromuscular strengthening is needed to attain the optimal 0.6–0.7 range.

These outcomes align with prior findings that highlight the therapeutic effects of hydrostatic pressure in reducing postoperative swelling and facilitating venous and lymphatic return (Buckthorpe et al., 2019). The early restoration of joint mobility observed in this case reinforces the argument that aquatic immersion can support more efficient oedema resolution and pain modulation than equivalent land-based strategies. This also reflects the biomechanical advantages identified by Prins and Cutner (1999), who emphasised the role of buoyancy and viscosity in reducing axial loading and enabling safe, graded resistance training, principles that underpinned the individual's early rehabilitation process.

Moreover, Peng (2023) demonstrated that aquatic therapy significantly improved range of motion, strength, and overall functional recovery in individuals with knee injuries, particularly among athletic populations. Echoing the present case, these findings affirm that structured aquatic programmes can promote muscular agility, reduce inflammation, and accelerate recovery when compared with passive or solely land-based approaches.

Affirmative Identity and Self-Determination

Psychological responses such as fear of re-injury, kinesiophobia, and emotional vulnerability are common following ACL injury (Flanigan et al., 2013; Little et al., 2023). In this case, the hydrotherapy setting provided a psychologically supportive and non-judgemental environment that fostered emotional resilience and a renewed sense of bodily agency. These experiences contributed to the individual's growing self-efficacy and capacity to engage meaningfully in movement without fear.

This process was reflected in a reduction in the individual's kinesiophobia score (TSK-11) from 35 to 25, indicating greater confidence in movement and a diminished fear response. Notably, the individual's Athletic Identity Measurement Scale (AIMS) score shifted from 50 pre-intervention to 41 post-intervention. Rather than representing a loss, this change marked an evolution from a narrowly defined, performance-based identity to a broader, more balanced self-concept, one that allowed for new expressions of physicality and strength.

These changes correspond with Subdimension 2a: Self-efficacy, and 2d: Resilience within the Four-Dimensional Model. The individual's narrative revealed a transition from anxiety and frustration toward increased confidence, adaptability, and emotional self-regulation. Hydrotherapy thus served not only as a means of physical recovery but also as a catalyst for identity redefinition and psychological empowerment.

Social Belonging and Inclusion

Although the early stages of intervention were delivered individually, the final phase integrated group-based aquatic activities that fostered peer connection and social engagement. Cooperative drills, such as paired agility tasks and resistance-band group challenges, created opportunities for shared effort, mutual encouragement, and enjoyment. These interactive elements supported not only physical coordination but also emotional attunement and interpersonal trust.

Such experiences align with Subdimension 3b: Group Cooperation and 3c: Belonging within the Four-Dimensional Model. The individual reported increased motivation and emotional uplift during group sessions, noting a renewed sense of being 'part of something', a shift from individual recovery to communal participation.

These findings are supported by research demonstrating that inclusive, group-based hydrotherapy enhances both engagement and psychosocial well-being (Martínez-Rodríguez et al., 2021; Pérez-de la Cruz, 2020). In this case, the group dynamic contributed meaningfully to the individual's sense of connectedness and reinforced their confidence through shared movement experiences in a supportive aquatic setting.

Holistic Well-Being and Long-Term Impact

Although the individual had not yet resumed competitive sport, he had successfully reintegrated into daily routines and light recreational activities. His progress reflects meaningful functional recovery, yet also underscores the importance of sustained attention to strength, proprioception, and psychological readiness in supporting long-term outcomes.

Beyond physical gains, the gradual recalibration of his athletic identity, shifting from an exclusive sport-centred self-concept to a broader and more balanced sense of self, points to a deeper form of recovery. Renewed motivation, physical confidence, and emotional resilience suggest that the hydrotherapy programme contributed not only to rehabilitation but also to personal adaptation and future-oriented well-being.

This case illustrates that long-term success in rehabilitation is not solely determined by performance thresholds, but by the individual's ability to reclaim agency, re-engage meaningfully with life, and sustain their own trajectory of health and identity development. These outcomes align closely with Subdimensions 4a: Functional Transfer, 4b: Quality of Life, and 4c: Health Behaviour Sustainability.

Conclusion

This case report illustrates the value of the Four-Dimensional Model of Hydrotherapy in supporting comprehensive rehabilitation following anterior cruciate ligament and meniscal injury. By extending beyond physical recovery to encompass identity formation, social inclusion, and long-term well-being, the model offers a person-centred framework for guiding practice and evaluating outcomes.

The case highlights hydrotherapy's potential to facilitate not only biomechanical progress but also psychological adaptation and renewed life engagement, particularly when injury disrupts core aspects of self-concept, autonomy, and everyday participation. These findings reinforce the importance of interdisciplinary, inclusive, and values-driven approaches to rehabilitation that recognise the individual as more than a site of injury, but as an active agent in their own recovery journey.

Participant Perspective[3]

Before my injury, soccer wasn't just something I did, it was who I was. My entire life revolved around training, competition, and the feeling of complete control over my body. Then, in a single moment, that was taken from me. After surgery, every step felt foreign, like my body no longer belonged to me. The worst part wasn't even the pain, it was the doubt. Would I ever feel like an athlete again? Would I ever trust my knee the way I used to?

At first, hydrotherapy felt like just another part of rehab, but I quickly realised it was different. In the water, I wasn't fragile. I could push myself, regain strength, and experiment with movement without fear of reinjury. The buoyancy let me test my limits safely, and as the sessions went on, I felt something I hadn't in a long time- control.

One of the biggest moments for me was when I started doing deep-water jumping drills. The first time, I hesitated. My mind immediately went to everything that could go wrong, the strain on my knee, the possibility of pain, the fear that my leg wouldn't hold up. But in the water, I had a second chance to trust my body again. The first jump was small, cautious. The second was stronger. By the end of the session, I wasn't just jumping- I was moving with confidence again. Working with others in the water, pushing each other to jump higher, move faster, showed me that I wasn't alone in this. The group dynamic made the exercises more engaging.

Then came the conversation with my orthopedic surgeon. He told me that while my recovery was going well, playing soccer at a high competitive level would put me at serious risk for another ACL injury, especially given the meniscus damage. That hit me hard. For months, I had been working toward the idea that I was going back to the exact version of myself I was before. But in that moment, I realised, I had already changed.

Hydrotherapy had taught me to move differently, to trust my body in new ways. Instead of thinking about what I had lost, I started thinking about what I had gained, better control, deeper awareness of my movement, and a new kind of athleticism that wasn't just about speed or power but about resilience and adaptability.

I won't be returning to the same soccer field I left behind, but I'm not leaving behind the athlete in me. Maybe I'll coach, maybe I'll compete in other ways, but what I know for sure is that my body is still strong. I am still strong. I don't need to chase who I was before, because I'm building something new, something just as powerful.[4]

A FOUR-DIMENSIONAL MODEL APPROACH TO HYDROTHERAPY REHABILITATION OF A 60-YEAR-OLD WOMAN WITH OSTEOARTHRITIS AND CHRONIC BACK PAIN USING AI CHI

Abstract

Background: Osteoarthritis (OA) and chronic back pain are highly prevalent among older adults, leading to pain, reduced mobility, and increased fall risk. Hydrotherapy, particularly Ai Chi, offers a low-impact, mindfulness-based intervention that may enhance functional outcomes and psychological well-being.

Case Presentation: A 60-year-old woman with bilateral knee and hip OA, chronic lower back pain, and a pronounced fear of falling reported declining physical activity, balance deficits, and progressive social withdrawal. Baseline assessments indicated impaired mobility (Timed Up and Go = 14.3 s), moderate fall risk (Berg Balance Scale = 40), and psychological impact (Tampa Scale of Kinesiophobia = 31; Geriatric Depression Scale = 7).

Intervention: The participant engaged in a 12-week, group-based Ai Chi hydrotherapy programme, delivered in three progressive phases: adaptation and pain reduction, strength and proprioceptive training, and transition to independent mobility. Sessions incorporated Ai Chi movement sequences, partnered balance exercises, and peer support strategies.

Outcomes: At follow-up, the participant demonstrated meaningful improvements: Timed Up and Go reduced to 11.8 s, Berg Balance Scale improved to 47, and Five-Times Sit-to-Stand Test improved to 12.5 s. Pain levels and kinesiophobia were reduced, and depressive symptoms improved (GDS = 4). Mild gait asymmetry persisted, and continued land-based strength training was recommended.

Conclusion: This case illustrates the multidimensional benefits of Ai Chi hydrotherapy for older adults with OA, addressing physical, emotional, and social dimensions of recovery. The Four-Dimensional Model of Hydrotherapy offered a structured framework for evaluating whole-person rehabilitation outcomes.

Keywords: Ai Chi, Balance, Case Report, Fear of Falling, Hydrotherapy, Osteoarthritis, Resilience

Introduction

Osteoarthritis (OA) is one of the most prevalent musculoskeletal conditions affecting older adults, particularly involving the hip and knee joints (Song & Oh, 2022). It is a degenerative joint disease characterised by cartilage degradation, bone remodelling, inflammation, and joint stiffness, which can lead to chronic pain, restricted mobility, and reduced quality of life (Franco et al., 2017). The persistent discomfort heightens fall risk and contribute to physical inactivity, which may further accelerate joint deterioration and compromise balance. Chronic lower back pain, frequently co-occurring with OA also affect postural control (Song & Oh, 2022).

Hydrotherapy has gained recognition as a valuable intervention for individuals with OA due to the unique therapeutic properties of water. Buoyancy reduces gravitational loading, facilitating movement with minimal joint strain, while hydrostatic pressure enhances circulation, decreases swelling, and improves proprioceptive feedback. Warm-water immersion promotes muscle relaxation, reduces stiffness, and increases joint range of motion- factors that together support improved function in older adults with musculoskeletal challenges (Franco et al., 2017; Song & Oh, 2022).

Ai Chi is a water-based movement technique that combines diaphragmatic breathing with slow, flowing postures to promote muscular control, postural stability, and relaxation (Lambeck & Bommer, 2010). Research suggests that Ai Chi enhances proprioception, balance, and fall prevention, particularly among individuals with postural instability (Kurt et al., 2018; Nissim et al., 2021). The method's emphasis on mindfulness and body awareness has also been associated with reduced fear of falling and improved confidence in movement.

This case report presents a structured hydrotherapy intervention using Ai Chi principles for a 60-year-old woman with knee and hip osteoarthritis, chronic back pain, and balance deficits. The rehabilitation process is analysed through the Four-Dimensional Model of Hydrotherapy, which evaluates outcomes across the following dimensions:

1. Body Functioning and Sensory Experience: Examining the physiological effects of Ai Chi on musculoskeletal function, proprioception, and pain modulation.
2. Affirmative Identity and Self-Determination: Exploring the impact of hydrotherapy on self-efficacy, autonomy, and psychological resilience.
3. Social Belonging and Inclusion: Assessing how hydrotherapy supports motivation, emotional well-being, and meaningful social participation.
4. Holistic Well-Being and Long-Term Impact: Evaluating the sustainability of outcomes and strategies for maintaining mobility and functional independence.

This approach aims to illustrate the integrative potential of hydrotherapy beyond conventional biomechanical models, reinforcing its value in promoting autonomy, participation, and well-being for adults living with OA and mobility-related challenges.

Participant Information[5]

A 60-year-old woman reported ongoing pain in both knees and hips, chronic lower back discomfort, and increasing difficulties with balance and walking. Over the previous three years, she had experienced a gradual decline in mobility, especially when navigating uneven surfaces, climbing stairs, or standing for extended periods. These changes led to reduced physical activity and growing social withdrawal. She began relying more heavily on a cane and expressed heightened anxiety about falling, often avoiding outdoor walking unless accompanied.

She was diagnosed with bilateral knee and hip osteoarthritis (OA) five years earlier, with imaging confirming joint space narrowing, osteophyte formation, and mild subchondral sclerosis. Alongside OA, she was managing mild osteoporosis and hypertension, treated with calcium and vitamin D supplementation and antihypertensive medication. Despite consistent adherence to a conservative treatment plan, comprising NSAIDs, intra-articular corticosteroid injections, and supervised land-based physiotherapy, her symptoms progressively worsened.

Beyond the physical challenges, she described growing frustration, lowered mood, and increasing withdrawal from social activities. While not formally diagnosed with depression, her score on the Geriatric Depression Scale (GDS) was 7, indicating mild psychological distress. She noted a reduction in independence, with daily tasks such as dressing, navigating stairs, and rising from a chair becoming more difficult. Her fear of falling strongly influenced her daily decisions, contributing to further avoidance of movement.

Prior to the onset of significant mobility limitations, she had led an active lifestyle and regularly enjoyed walking. However, as pain and apprehension intensified, she gradually reduced her structured physical activity.

Health and Functional Profile[6]

A comprehensive physical assessment identified bilateral knee crepitus, joint effusion, and tenderness along both the medial and lateral joint lines. Passive range of motion was moderately limited, with knee flexion restricted to 110° bilaterally and reduced internal rotation at the hips- findings consistent with age-related joint degeneration. Manual muscle testing indicated mild-to-moderate weakness in the quadriceps and gluteal muscles. Dynamic balance assessments revealed instability during single-leg stance and tandem walking.

Her score on the Berg Balance Scale (BBS) was 40/56, indicating a moderate risk of falling. On the Timed Up and Go (TUG) test, she recorded 14.3 seconds – above the 13.5-second cut-off for increased fall risk in older adults. Her Five-Times Sit-to-Stand Test result exceeded 15 seconds, reflecting reduced lower-limb strength and difficulty transitioning between seated and standing positions.

Gait analysis showed a reduced walking speed of 0.8 metres per second, a shortened stride length of 0.72 metres, and asymmetric weight-bearing, with greater reliance on her non-dominant leg. Postural analysis revealed increased anterior pelvic tilt and compensatory lumbar lordosis.

Her Tampa Scale of Kinesiophobia (TSK-11) score was 31, suggesting significant movement-related fear, which further impacted her confidence and willingness to remain active. Pain levels were rated as 6/10 at rest and 8/10 during movement using the Visual Analogue Scale (VAS). Her BMI, recorded at 30.1kg/m^2, placed her in the clinical obesity category, a recognised factor in osteoarthritis progression.

Radiographic imaging confirmed moderate-to-severe osteoarthritis, with marked joint space narrowing – particularly in the medial compartments of the knees. Additional findings included osteophyte formation in both the femorotibial and femoroacetabular joints, as well as mild subchondral sclerosis, indicating progressive cartilage degeneration. MRI was not deemed necessary, as the radiographic findings adequately explained her clinical presentation.

Previous interventions had included corticosteroid injections, which offered only short-term relief, and multiple cycles of land-based physiotherapy. However, ongoing difficulties with proprioception and movement confidence limited the long-term benefits of these approaches. In view of her balance concerns, increasing functional limitations, and fear of falling, a structured hydrotherapy programme was recommended to support safer movement, enhance functional capacity, and promote overall well-being.

Therapeutic Intervention

A structured, 12-week Ai Chi hydrotherapy programme was introduced to promote mobility, postural stability, and holistic well-being. The intervention was delivered in a group format comprising eight participants, with sessions conducted twice weekly in a warm-water therapy pool maintained at 33°C. Each session lasted approximately 40 minutes.

The programme followed a progressive structure, combining core Ai Chi movement sequences with functional mobility and balance training. The slow, flowing movements, synchronised with deep diaphragmatic breathing, were selected to support dynamic postural control, reduce joint loading, and enhance sensory-motor integration. As the sessions progressed, the exercises were gradually adapted to reflect each participant's capabilities, allowing for individual variation within the group setting.

The warm, supportive aquatic environment enabled movement with minimal discomfort and created a psychologically safe space in which participants could explore new movement strategies without fear of falling. The integration of structured group activity also provided opportunities for peer encouragement and shared engagement, fostering emotional motivation and social connection alongside physical recovery.

Phase 1: Adaptation and Pain Reduction (Weeks 1–4)

The initial phase focused on acclimatising participants to the aquatic environment, reducing pain and stiffness, and fostering confidence in supported movement. This stage employed Ai Chi exclusively, offering a structured, gradual introduction to water immersion, proprioceptive awareness, and postural control. The slow, flowing movements were selected to support adaptation to hydrostatic pressure, breath regulation, and neuromuscular coordination, while cultivating a sense of safety in the aquatic setting.

The first five Ai Chi movements formed the foundation of this phase, each intentionally aligned with specific hydrodynamic properties to promote adaptation and functional readiness:

1. Contemplating: Centred on deep diaphragmatic breathing, this movement activated the parasympathetic nervous system, promoting muscle relaxation and pain modulation through buoyancy-assisted breath synchronisation.
2. Floating: Involved slow, controlled upper-limb movements to stimulate proprioceptive input and encourage progressive postural relaxation under hydrostatic pressure.
3. Uplifting: Introduced vertical hand movements synchronised with exhalation, supporting venous return and gradual postural realignment.
4. Enclosing: Integrated fluid scapular motion, enhancing postural awareness and facilitating safe movement exposure essential for developing confidence in dynamic balance.
5. Folding: Reinforced neuromuscular coordination while minimising articular loading, offering a low-impact route to joint mobility enhancement.

Movements were performed in a semi-flexed standing posture to provide a stable base of support while adjusting to water viscosity and resistance. A group-based format was intentionally used to promote peer encouragement and relational engagement, contributing to emotional safety and social motivation.

Each session concluded with a brief guided reflection, allowing participants to articulate bodily sensations, progress, or concerns. These discussions reinforced a sense of shared experience and laid the psychosocial groundwork for further therapeutic progression.

Phase 2: Strength and Proprioceptive Training (Weeks 5–8)

As the intervention progressed, the emphasis shifted toward enhancing muscular strength, proprioceptive control, and postural stability, while continuing to build psychological readiness for more dynamic movement. Ai Chi sequences were expanded to incorporate coordinated, full-body patterns, integrating the subsequent ten movements: Soothing, Gathering, Accepting, Freeing, Shifting, Presenting, Opening, Encircling, Flowing, and Reflecting. These exercises were performed in synchrony to promote rhythmic flow, neuromuscular coordination, and a shared sense of engagement within the group.

Participants were guided to move with intention and control, using the natural resistance of water to develop muscular endurance and trunk stabilisation while maintaining joint alignment. The meditative pace of Ai Chi continued to support emotional regulation and attentional focus, key elements in rebuilding confidence in movement.

To further challenge dynamic balance and sensory integration, Ne Ai Chi (partnered Ai Chi) was introduced. This practice involved mirroring movements with a partner, offering tactile feedback and promoting interpersonal attunement. The reciprocal nature of Ne Ai Chi strengthened proprioceptive responsiveness and enhanced awareness of body positioning in space.

Controlled perturbation drills were also introduced, incorporating gentle water turbulence or partner-assisted resistance to activate core stabilisers and refine equilibrium responses. These activities simulated real-world balance challenges in a safe, graded manner.

Sessions were accompanied by calming background music to reinforce relaxation and rhythm, fostering a mind-body connection. By the end of this phase, participants demonstrated improved postural control in the aquatic environment, reduced apprehension during movement transitions, and greater confidence in engaging with complex movement patterns. These outcomes prepared the group for more functional and task-specific activity in the final phase.

Phase 3: Transition to Independent Mobility (Weeks 9–12)

The final phase of the programme centred on strengthening functional mobility, promoting autonomous engagement in physical activity, and supporting the transition to sustained community participation. Each session commenced with a full sequence of Ai Chi movements, reinforcing fluidity, postural alignment, and confidence in progressively weight-bearing environments.

To simulate real-life mobility demands, participants practised stepping over low obstacles, ascending and descending simulated kerbs, and performing multidirectional walking drills. These activities were conducted in progressively shallower water, gradually increasing gravitational loading while maintaining postural support and joint safety. The shift from deep to shallower immersion served to enhance neuromuscular readiness for land-based movement and functional independence.

Social belonging and peer reinforcement were key themes in this phase. Group-based Ai Chi circles encouraged synchronised movement and subtle balance adaptation, fostering shared rhythm and mutual responsiveness. Participants engaged in peer-led sequences, where individuals guided selected movements while others followed, promoting leadership, movement autonomy, and self-efficacy. These experiences contributed to advancing subdimension 2a: Self-efficacy and 3b: Group cooperation within the Four-Dimensional Model.

To support long-term behavioural sustainability, structured group discussions were integrated at the close of each session. These conversations invited participants to reflect on their personal progress, share coping strategies, and consider how Ai Chi could be maintained as a regular wellness practice beyond the formal intervention. Topics included identifying accessible community resources, creating home-based routines, and using audio or video guidance to reinforce learned sequences. These discussions deepened emotional engagement and reinforced motivation for continued participation.

The facilitator highlighted the availability of community-based aquatic groups and emphasised the psychological and physical benefits of ongoing involvement. During structured group discussions participants reported enhanced confidence, reduced fear of falling, improved coordination, and renewed motivation to remain active.

By integrating mindful movement, task-specific training, and group cohesion, this phase reinforced both the functional transfer (subdimension 4a) and health behaviour sustainability (subdimension 4c) elements of the model. The programme concluded with participants expressing their intentions to remain engaged with aquatic practice, viewing Ai Chi not only as a rehabilitative technique but as a lifelong resource for independence, emotional regulation, and fall prevention.

Follow-up and Outcomes

At the 12-week follow-up, the individual exhibited meaningful improvements in balance, functional mobility, pain modulation, and psychological resilience. These gains, while notable, were accompanied by residual limitations in land-based strength and gait adaptability, suggesting the need for continued intervention to consolidate progress and promote long-term autonomy.

Functional mobility improved, with the Timed Up and Go (TUG) score decreasing from 14.3 to 11.8 seconds – a change indicating reduced fall risk and enhanced dynamic movement capacity. Nonetheless, the individual continued to express mild apprehension when navigating stairs or walking unaided over uneven surfaces, reflecting lingering movement-related anxiety.

Balance assessment revealed a Berg Balance Scale (BBS) improvement from 40 to 47, signifying greater postural control, particularly in transitional tasks such as standing from a seated position and tandem stance. However, occasional challenges in reactive balance, especially in unpredictable environments, highlighted areas for further skill development in postural adjustment and confidence under dynamic conditions.

Pain levels showed moderate reduction, with Visual Analogue Scale (VAS) scores declining from 8/10 to 6/10 during activity, and from 6/10 to 4/10 at rest. The warm-water environment, hydrostatic compression, and supportive movement practice were instrumental in alleviating stiffness and increasing comfort. Nevertheless, discomfort persisted following prolonged standing or repetitive weight-bearing tasks, emphasising the importance of continued joint care and tailored activity pacing.

Lower-limb strength improved as evidenced by a reduction in the Five-Times Sit-to-Stand test time, from over 15 seconds to 12.5 seconds, indicating better quadriceps and gluteal endurance. While aquatic resistance contributed to this improvement, land-based endurance and muscular power remained areas requiring further focus, particularly in weight-bearing activities such as stair climbing or prolonged walking.

Gait analysis revealed progress in stride length and walking velocity; however, asymmetry persisted, with continued reliance on the non-dominant leg during loading tasks. These findings pointed to a need for targeted gait retraining in gravity-dependent settings to improve symmetry and movement efficiency.

Psychologically, the Tampa Scale of Kinesiophobia (TSK-11) score decreased from 31 to 22, suggesting a reduction in movement-related fear and greater willingness to engage with physical activity. The group-based Ai Chi environment contributed to this shift by offering graded exposure, rhythmical movement, and peer reassurance. Nonetheless, the individual reported ongoing caution in navigating crowded environments, indicating the value of extended community practice to reinforce confidence.

In terms of mood and social well-being, the Geriatric Depression Scale (GDS) score improved from 7 to 4, indicating a reduction in low mood and social withdrawal. The structured, peer-supported nature of the programme fostered interpersonal connection, emotional safety, and renewed motivation, advancing the subdimensions of 3c: Belonging and 4b: Quality of Life.

A transition plan was developed to support continued progress. The individual was encouraged to participate in community-based Ai Chi or aquatic wellness groups, and to gradually incorporate land-based strengthening exercises tailored to her needs. These recommendations aimed to support functional transfer (4a) and health behaviour sustainability (4c), reinforcing the long-term benefits of the hydrotherapy experience.

Overall, this case illustrates how a group-based Ai Chi intervention can promote meaningful gains in mobility, pain management, psychological well-being, and social connection for older adults managing osteoarthritis and balance-related challenges. While full functional independence was not yet achieved, the structured support of the programme laid the groundwork for continued engagement, emotional resilience, and adaptive physical confidence.

Discussion

The rehabilitation of older adults with osteoarthritis (OA) and mobility impairments requires a multidimensional approach that extends beyond biomechanical restoration, encompassing physical function, psychological adaptation, social participation, and long-term well-being. Aquatic interventions offer distinct advantages by leveraging the properties of water, buoyancy, hydrostatic pressure, and thermotherapy, to reduce joint loading and promote functional movement (Song & Oh, 2022).

This case study explored the outcomes of a structured 12-week Ai Chi hydrotherapy programme delivered in a group format for a 60-year-old woman with bilateral knee and hip OA, chronic lower back pain, and progressive gait instability. The intervention was examined through the lens of the Four-Dimensional Model of Hydrotherapy, which integrates the domains of Body Functioning and Sensory Experience, Affirmative Identity and Self-Determination, Social Belonging and Inclusion, and Holistic Well-Being and Long-Term Impact.

Body Functioning and Sensory Experience

The participant experienced meaningful improvements in functional mobility, balance, and pain modulation, in line with previous research highlighting the value of hydrotherapy in supporting individuals with OA (Song & Oh, 2022; Lambeck & Bommer, 2010). Warm-water immersion contributed to enhanced joint mobility and a reduction in stiffness, while the structured, flowing movements of Ai Chi supported proprioceptive awareness and neuromuscular coordination. These outcomes reflect broader findings from meta-analytic studies indicating that aquatic exercise is associated with pain reduction and improved joint function in populations with osteoarthritis (Song & Oh, 2022).

Functionally, the participant's Berg Balance Scale (BBS) score increased from 40 to 47, and her Timed Up and Go (TUG) performance improved from 14.3 to 11.8 seconds, reflecting enhanced postural control and reduced fall risk. These results align with prior evidence supporting the use of aquatic therapy to improve mobility outcomes among individuals with OA (Hinman et al., 2007). Notably, given that previous trials have reported modest improvements in TUG scores, the extent of progress observed here may be attributed to the sustained duration of the programme and the integrative use of Ai Chi techniques. While these gains were encouraging, the presence of residual gait asymmetry and ongoing weight-bearing limitations highlights the need for continued proprioceptive training and land-based strength support to further consolidate mobility gains.

Affirmative Identity and Self-Determination

Psychological experiences, particularly fear of movement and reduced confidence in mobility, play a significant role in influencing rehabilitation engagement and outcomes (Flanigan et al., 2013; Ohji et al., 2021). At baseline, the participant reported a high level of movement-related fear, reflected in a TSK-11 score of 31, which suggested notable apprehension and avoidance behaviour. By the conclusion of the programme, her score had decreased to 22, indicating a meaningful reduction in fear-avoidance patterns and an increase in her confidence to engage in movement.

The adaptable, gentle structure of Ai Chi directly supported subdimensions 2a (self-efficacy) and 2d (resilience), by cultivating embodied awareness and reinforcing the participant's sense of autonomy and capacity for self-directed progress. These observations are in line with previous findings suggesting that Ai Chi enhances self-efficacy among older adults by providing a safe, affirming environment that encourages gradual re-engagement with movement (Lambeck & Bommer, 2010).

Although the participant expressed a renewed willingness to engage in structured activity, she remained somewhat hesitant in crowded or unpredictable environments, preferring to retain the use of an assistive device. This cautious approach may indicate the need for additional opportunities to practise mobility tasks in land-based settings, in order to further consolidate her confidence and readiness for fully independent movement.

Social Belonging and Inclusion

Supportive social interaction is widely recognised as a key factor in promoting both engagement with rehabilitation and psychological well-being among older adults (Martínez-Rodríguez et al., 2021). Within the group-based Ai Chi sessions, participants experienced a sense of shared purpose, mutual encouragement, and emotional resonance, which contributed to a more positive and affirming rehabilitation environment. The participant's Geriatric Depression Scale (GDS) score improved from 7 to 4, suggesting a reduction in emotional distress and social withdrawal.

The synchronised movement sequences advanced subdimension 3c (belonging), transforming individual movement into a meaningful group experience. This finding echoes evidence that aquatic group interventions can enhance motivation, increase participation, and improve perceived quality of life for individuals living with osteoarthritis (Song & Oh, 2022). In addition, the inclusion of guided group discussions after sessions provided space for reflection, peer learning, and connection, further supporting emotional safety and long-term engagement.

The participant expressed a renewed sense of agency in how she navigated her environment and interacted with others, highlighting the importance of group-based formats not only for physical rehabilitation, but also for fostering emotional support, shared motivation, and a sense of social connection. These relational aspects are particularly important in sustaining long-term physical activity and preventing isolation, which can significantly impact quality of life in later adulthood.

Holistic Well-Being and Long-Term Impact

Supporting individuals to sustain progress beyond the formal rehabilitation period is essential for promoting lasting well-being and reducing the risk of functional decline in people living with osteoarthritis. While the participant in this case experienced meaningful improvements in mobility, pain levels, and psychological resilience, some challenges remained, particularly in weight-bearing symmetry and endurance. Gait analysis revealed a continued reliance on the non-dominant leg, highlighting the importance of ongoing support to strengthen movement confidence and physical capacity in everyday contexts.

Long-term engagement in structured physical activity is a key factor in maintaining health gains, yet research suggests that aquatic exercise on its own may not fully support muscular strength over time (Song & Oh, 2022). To address this, a personalised transition plan was offered, incorporating continued Ai Chi participation within a community-based setting, alongside progressive land-based strength training. This blended approach is supported by evidence showing that integrating hydrotherapy with neuromuscular conditioning leads to more sustainable outcomes in individuals with OA (Song & Oh, 2022).

Given the social and emotional benefits the participant described during the group programme, connecting with peer-led aquatic groups was also encouraged as a way to reinforce motivation, reduce isolation, and promote long-term adherence. To support adaptive progression, periodic reassessment of balance and mobility was recommended, ensuring that emerging challenges can be addressed proactively. Together, these strategies support the continuity of person-centred care, reinforcing not only physical function, but also autonomy, confidence, and sustained engagement in meaningful activity.

Conclusion

This case study highlights the multidimensional role of Ai Chi hydrotherapy in OA rehabilitation, demonstrating its benefits across physical, psychological, social, and long-term well-being domains. The Four-Dimensional Model of Hydrotherapy provided a structured framework for assessing the intervention's impact beyond biomechanical recovery, reinforcing the importance of self-efficacy, social engagement, and holistic rehabilitation strategies.

While the individual experienced notable improvements in balance, mobility, and psychological resilience, the persistence of gait asymmetries and weight-bearing challenges underscores the need for continued strength training and access to community-based movement programmes. These findings support the integration of person-centred aquatic interventions into rehabilitation services for older adults, and underscore the importance of health policies that promote inclusive, sustainable, and socially engaging approaches to ageing well.

Participant Perspective[7]

When I first started hydrotherapy, I was sceptical. I had tried so many different treatments, pain medication, physiotherapy, even corticosteroid injections, but nothing provided lasting relief. My knees and hips were always stiff, my back ached constantly, and I was always afraid of falling. Walking outside, especially on uneven surfaces, became something I avoided unless someone was with me.

At first, I didn't understand how moving in water could help me. I worried that I would lose my balance, struggle to follow the movements, or feel self-conscious in front of others. But after a few sessions, something unexpected happened, the movement felt easier. On land, every step felt heavy and painful, but in the water, I could shift my weight, move my legs, and stretch without the same level of discomfort.

One of the biggest changes for me was how I started to feel about movement itself. Before, I was so afraid of falling that I avoided walking too much. But in the pool, I could challenge my balance without fear. The slow, flowing movements of Ai Chi helped me reconnect with my body, and over time, I noticed my confidence improving.

But more than anything, the water gave me relief, not just from the pain, but from the heaviness I feel every day. How wonderful it would be if our whole lives could be spent in water. Everything would feel so much easier.[8]

A FOUR-DIMENSIONAL MODEL APPROACH TO HYDROTHERAPY WITH A 14-YEAR-OLD BOY WITH QUADRIPLEGIC CEREBRAL PALSY AND CORTICAL VISUAL IMPAIRMENT: A HALLIWICK CONCEPT CASE REPORT

Abstract

Background: A 12-week Halliwick-based hydrotherapy programme was implemented to support a young person with quadriplegic cerebral palsy (QCP) and cortical visual impairment (CVI) in enhancing movement, sensory integration, and participation in everyday life. QCP and CVI can affect motor coordination, spatial orientation, and access to physical activity. The Halliwick Concept offers a structured aquatic framework that promotes motor learning, autonomy, and social engagement in a safe and inclusive environment. The Four-Dimensional Model of Hydrotherapy provides a person-centred lens for evaluating progress beyond biomechanical outcomes.

Case Presentation: The participant, a 14-year-old boy who uses a power wheelchair and requires full assistance with activities of daily living, engaged in weekly hydrotherapy sessions. He had an established therapeutic relationship with a consistent hydrotherapist and experienced anxiety in unfamiliar settings. Baseline assessments indicated profound motor limitations (GMFM-66: 12.8), elevated muscle tone (MAS Grade 3), and pain rated 6/10 (FLACC scale).

Intervention: Over 12 weeks, the individual participated in Halliwick-based sessions incorporating floating, rotational control, auditory-guided propulsion, and cooperative aquatic tasks. Warm-water conditions (33 °C) supported relaxation and reduced discomfort. Activities were designed to foster movement confidence, postural control, and self-directed mobility, while group components encouraged communication and peer interaction.

Outcomes: At follow-up, improvements were observed across multiple domains: GMFM-66 score increased to 18.4, pain reduced to 3/10, and the participant achieved five metres of independent propulsion using flippers. He demonstrated increased openness to working with different facilitators and enhanced social engagement with peers. While fatigue and sensitivity to environmental unpredictability remained, a structured transition plan was developed to support sustained aquatic participation and inclusion in adapted swimming activities.

Conclusion: This case illustrates the multidimensional benefits of a Halliwick-based hydrotherapy approach for a young person with complex motor and sensory needs. Notable gains were achieved in mobility, self-efficacy, and social participation. The Four-Dimensional Model of Hydrotherapy provided a valuable framework for holistic assessment, encompassing functional ability, emotional well-being, community inclusion, and long-term potential. Continued access to warm-water, disability-inclusive settings is essential to support ongoing engagement and well-being.

Keywords: Cerebral Palsy, Cortical Visual Impairment, Four-Dimensional Model of Hydrotherapy, Halliwick Concept, Paediatric Rehabilitation, Person-Centred Practice.

Introduction

Cerebral palsy (CP) is a non-progressive neurological condition that affects movement, posture, and muscle tone. Quadriplegic cerebral palsy (QCP), a subtype of CP, is characterised by motor disability in all four limbs and is often accompanied by spasticity, dystonia, and co-occurring conditions such as epilepsy, orthopaedic complications, and cortical visual impairment (CVI) (Viswanath et al., 2023; Vova, 2022). CVI, the leading cause of visual impairment in children, affects the brain's ability to process visual information, resulting in difficulties with contrast sensitivity, depth perception, and spatial orientation (Mohapatra et al., 2022). These combined motor and sensory challenges significantly limit mobility, communication, and participation in everyday life, requiring a comprehensive, multidisciplinary rehabilitation approach that addresses physical, sensory, and functional dimensions.

Hydrotherapy has been recognised as an effective intervention for children with CP, making use of the unique properties of water, buoyancy, resistance, and hydrostatic pressure, to facilitate movement, enhance postural control, and promote engagement in physical activity (Xiang et al., 2024). In addition to its physical benefits, hydrotherapy offers a socially inclusive and emotionally supportive environment that can foster participation, communication, and self-expression. The Halliwick Concept is a structured aquatic therapy approach designed to promote motor learning, dynamic balance, and independence in the water. It is particularly well suited for individuals with QCP, as it emphasises breath control, relaxation, and rotational movement skills, supporting the development of safe and functional aquatic mobility (Gajić et al., 2020).

The Four-Dimensional Model of Hydrotherapy offers a structured, multidimensional framework for evaluating outcomes in aquatic rehabilitation that extend beyond biomechanical recovery:

1. Body Functioning and Sensory Experience: Examines the impact of hydrotherapy on postural alignment, muscle coordination, and sensory integration.
2. Affirmative Identity and Self-Determination: Explores how water-based interventions foster self-confidence, emotional regulation, and a sense of autonomy.
3. Social Belonging and Inclusion: Assesses the extent to which aquatic sessions support communication, peer interaction, and meaningful group participation.
4. Holistic Well-Being and Long-Term Impact: Evaluates sustained improvements in physical activity, quality of life, and the integration of skills into everyday routines.

This case report presents the rehabilitation journey of a 14-year-old boy with QCP and CVI, who engaged in a Halliwick-based hydrotherapy programme. The intervention is analysed through the lens of the Four-Dimensional Model of Hydrotherapy, highlighting progress in aquatic independence, postural control, and psychosocial engagement, and demonstrating the broader therapeutic potential of hydrotherapy in supporting the holistic development of young people with complex disabilities.

Participant Information[9]

The participant is a 14-year-old boy attending a special education school that supports pupils with complex motor disabilities. He has a diagnosis of quadriplegic cerebral palsy (Gross Motor Function Classification System – GMFCS Level V) and cortical visual impairment (CVI), with residual vision limited to light perception and shadow detection. He is cognitively capable and verbally expressive, actively participating in classroom discussions and social interactions with both peers and staff.

He has taken part in weekly hydrotherapy sessions since infancy, beginning at the age of one. Early sessions were marked by heightened anxiety and avoidance behaviours, necessitating a gradual desensitisation approach and consistent exposure to the aquatic setting. Over time, he developed increased comfort in the water, though he continues to rely heavily on continuity of care. In the absence of his regular hydrotherapist, he typically declines to enter the pool, highlighting the importance of therapeutic rapport and predictability in his rehabilitation experience.

Transfers into the water are performed using a mechanical hoist, as he requires full assistance with mobility and personal care. He uses a powered wheelchair with a custom-moulded seating system providing pelvic and thoracic support, head positioning, and pressure relief to prevent pressure ulcers. He is fully dependent on caregivers for transfers, positioning, and activities of daily living. Upper limb function is significantly limited, with minimal selective motor control and pronounced spasticity affecting both fine and gross motor coordination.

Health and Functional Profile[10]

The participant was born prematurely at 28 weeks' gestation and was subsequently diagnosed with periventricular leukomalacia (PVL). His medical history includes well-controlled epilepsy, bilateral hip subluxation, and scoliosis, all of which are regularly monitored by his orthopaedic team. He also experiences recurrent respiratory infections, likely associated with reduced mobility and a diminished cough reflex. Due to severe dysphagia, all nutrition and hydration are administered via gastrostomy.

To support comfort and facilitate passive movement, the participant receives routine botulinum toxin injections targeting both upper and lower limbs to manage increased muscle tone. He engages in a comprehensive, interdisciplinary therapy programme, which includes:

- Physiotherapy: focusing on maintaining joint mobility and preventing contractures.
- Occupational therapy: supporting the use of assistive devices and promoting adaptations for limited fine motor control.
- Speech and language therapy: emphasising the development and refinement of augmentative and alternative communication (AAC) strategies to complement his verbal communication and support expressive language use.

Pre-intervention assessments highlighted significant motor challenges. His Gross Motor Function Measure (GMFM-66) score was 12.8/100, indicating very limited voluntary motor function. Muscle tone, evaluated using the Modified Ashworth Scale (MAS), was recorded at Grade 3 in all four limbs, with greater spasticity noted in the lower extremities. Pain was assessed via the FLACC scale and rated at 6/10, particularly during prolonged static positioning or passive range-of-motion exercises.

Therapeutic Intervention

A structured 12-week hydrotherapy programme based on the Halliwick Concept was implemented to promote functional mobility, support autonomy in aquatic environments, and encourage long-term participation in swimming as a physical activity. The intervention integrated systematic skill development, relational engagement, and personalised aquatic tasks, in accordance with the Halliwick Ten-Point Programme and the Four-Dimensional Model of Hydrotherapy.

Sessions were held once a week for 30 minutes in a warm-water therapy pool maintained at 33°C. The programme sought to enhance movement variability, counteract the sedentary effects of prolonged wheelchair use, and build confidence in aquatic movement. Beyond its rehabilitative aims, the intervention was also designed to cultivate swimming as a source of enjoyment, belonging, and lifelong engagement.

Phase 1: Foundational Mobility and Confidence Building (Weeks 1–4)

The initial phase focused on broadening the individual's repertoire of aquatic movements beyond passive floating, with an emphasis on dynamic postural transitions and early-stage social engagement within a supportive group setting. Given his prior experience with hydrotherapy, the intervention prioritised increasing movement variability and refining body control.

Core stability and trunk activation were promoted through active floating drills, incorporating lateral weight shifts and rotational transitions. Longitudinal and transverse rotation exercises supported the development of midline orientation and spatial awareness.

Propulsion training was introduced using modified backstroke movements with flippers, accompanied by auditory wayfinding cues to accommodate the individual's cortical visual impairment and strengthen spatial orientation. The transition from therapist-assisted to self-initiated movement was supported through structured confidence-building activities embedded in peer interaction. Cooperative floating tasks and group navigation exercises, such as "Follow the Sound", in which the individual oriented towards a peer's voice, reinforced self-confidence and directional control within a socially meaningful context.

Phase 2: Movement Initiation and Peer-Based Engagement (Weeks 5–8)

The second phase focused on enhancing the individual's capacity to initiate movement independently, promoting aquatic autonomy and expanding opportunities for peer-based interaction. Therapeutic support was progressively reduced to encourage self-reliance, and modified breaststroke kicking patterns were introduced to support bilateral lower-limb coordination.

Trunk control and anti-gravity postural stability were further developed through resisted floating drills designed to engage core musculature and reinforce midline orientation. Functional lower-limb movements, including hip extension and controlled kicking sequences, were integrated to facilitate volitional control and reduce spasticity.

Peer-led aquatic challenges, such as relay-style activities, incorporated verbal and tactile cues to promote communication, shared engagement, and collaborative goal pursuit. Obstacle navigation tasks were embedded to stimulate spatial reasoning, directional control, and adaptive motor planning in a safe and supportive aquatic context. Guided propulsion sequences continued to reinforce movement confidence, contributing to the gradual transition toward independent mobility with minimal therapeutic facilitation.

Phase 3: Transition to Long-Term Aquatic Participation (Weeks 9–12)

The final phase focused on consolidating functional progress and facilitating a transition towards sustained participation in aquatic activity beyond the structured therapeutic setting. Independent propulsion techniques were refined, with emphasis on stroke efficiency, breath control, and endurance. Structured interval training was introduced to enhance cardiovascular capacity within the constraints of the individual's motor abilities and respiratory function.

To promote psychological ownership of movement, the individual engaged in reflective goal-setting, identifying meaningful swimming milestones and articulating personal progress. These activities aimed to reinforce self-efficacy and intrinsic motivation for continued aquatic engagement. Adaptive swimming strategies were explored to prepare for potential participation in inclusive leisure or recreational programmes, ensuring alignment with the individual's preferences and abilities.

Peer-supported group activities remained a core element, promoting relational learning and social participation. The individual was invited to complete a self-evaluation task, involving independent propulsion over a set aquatic distance, reinforcing autonomy and marking a tangible personal achievement.

Follow-up and Outcomes

At the 12-week follow-up, the individual demonstrated meaningful improvements in aquatic mobility, postural control, and psychosocial engagement. While his underlying physical disability remained, he showed greater confidence and functional participation in the water, aligning with the broader rehabilitation goal of maintaining abilities and preventing further functional decline.

His capacity to initiate and modulate movement in the aquatic environment improved notably. He demonstrated enhanced transitions between floating and propulsion and exhibited increased tolerance for dynamic postural challenges. Of particular significance was his improved willingness to work with different hydrotherapists and engage with peers, reflecting a positive shift in trust, adaptability, and social interaction. This was especially meaningful given his longstanding reliance on therapeutic consistency and routine.

Functional assessments pre- and post-intervention indicated moderate, yet relevant, gains. His Gross Motor Function Measure (GMFM-66) score increased from 12.8 to 18.4, reflecting improved trunk control, movement variability, and participation in supported aquatic tasks. Although muscle tone remained at Grade 3 on the Modified Ashworth Scale, observable gains were evident in trunk stability and bilateral lower-limb propulsion during facilitated movement sequences. Pain, assessed via the FLACC scale, decreased from 6 to 3, suggesting improved comfort during prolonged positioning, likely attributable to enhanced muscular relaxation and increased joint mobility in the warm water setting.

The individual also demonstrated a marked improvement in independent propulsion. Whereas at baseline he required continuous physical guidance and verbal cueing, by week 12 he was able to propel himself using flippers for a distance of up to five metres, responding to auditory navigation cues provided by therapists and peers. Although endurance remained limited and fatigue occurred after brief activity, this level of functional movement represents a clinically meaningful progression in neuromuscular control and self-directed engagement.

Given the sensitivity of spasticity to temperature, it was recommended that aquatic participation continue in a hydrotherapeutic environment with controlled water temperature between 32°C and 34°C. Standard public pools were deemed unsuitable due to the risk of cold exposure and sensory overload. Structured adaptive swimming programmes in disability-inclusive facilities were identified as optimal for supporting long-term participation.

To maintain and expand on the progress made, a personalised transition plan was developed. This included continued hydrotherapy with progressive endurance training, group-based swimming sessions to reinforce social belonging and motivation, ongoing use of auditory wayfinding strategies to support spatial navigation, and gradual reduction in hands-on therapist support to encourage autonomy and self-initiated movement.

For individuals with complex disabilities, the primary aims of hydrotherapy are not full independence but rather preservation of function, enhancement of movement potential, and support for emotional well-being. The reduction in pain, expansion of movement repertoire, and increased social participation observed in this case underscore the value of hydrotherapy as a central component in holistic, multidisciplinary care.

Discussion

Rehabilitation for children with QCP and CVI requires a multidimensional, inclusive approach that addresses not only physical impairments but also sensory processing, emotional well-being, and meaningful participation. While land-based physiotherapy remains a cornerstone for people with cerebral palsy, hydrotherapy presents distinctive opportunities to enhance motor variability, promote sensory integration, and foster self-determined engagement in movement.

This case study examined the outcomes of a structured Halliwick-based hydrotherapy programme through the lens of the Four-Dimensional Model of Hydrotherapy. By evaluating progress across the dimensions of Body Functioning and Sensory Experience, Affirmative Identity and Self-Determination, Social Belonging and Inclusion, and Holistic Well-Being and Long-Term Impact, the case highlights how aquatic interventions can support whole-person development and sustained participation for children with complex physical and sensory needs.

Body Functioning and Sensory Experience

The Halliwick Concept's emphasis on motor learning, breath control, postural adjustment, and sensory adaptation makes it especially relevant for children with complex motor disabilities such as QCP (Lambeck & Gamper, 2011). In this case, the participant demonstrated clinically meaningful improvements in water-based movement control, as indicated by an increase in his GMFM-66 score from 12.8 to 18.4. Although muscle tone remained elevated (Modified Ashworth Scale Grade 3), he exhibited enhanced postural control and dynamic balance in the water, particularly during rotational transitions and lower-limb propulsion.

These gains reflect the supportive properties of the aquatic environment, which facilitate active movement and neuromuscular engagement without excessive gravitational strain (Gajić et al., 2020). The warm water (33°C) further contributed to reduced discomfort, with the FLACC pain score decreasing from 6/10 to 3/10. This underscores the importance of a thermally regulated pool setting for children with spasticity, as exposure to cooler water may increase muscle stiffness and reduce mobility efficiency (Becker, 2009). Together, these outcomes highlight the capacity of hydrotherapy to optimise sensory-motor functioning while minimising pain and fatigue in children with physical disabilities.

Affirmative Identity and Self-Determination

Hydrotherapy also served as a platform for fostering autonomy, self-efficacy, and psychological resilience. At baseline, the participant exhibited hesitancy when initiating movement, relying on continuous therapist support. Through the structured withdrawal of assistance, a core principle of the Halliwick Concept, he progressed to self-initiated back propulsion using auditory cues, reflecting meaningful gains in the subdimension of Self-efficacy within the Affirmative Identity and Self-Determination dimension. By week 12, he demonstrated the ability to propel himself independently for short distances, marking a meaningful shift in perceived agency and control.

These developments resonate with prior studies indicating that water-based interventions can reduce kinesiophobia and support self-determined physical activity in children with disabilities (Gajić et al., 2020). The transition from passive to active participation was not only functional but also symbolic, reflecting a redefinition of identity from 'dependent' to 'capable'. This shift is critical for young people with multiple disabilities, as it reinforces internal motivation and emotional well-being within the therapeutic process.

Social Belonging and Inclusion

Social engagement emerged as a vital dimension of the intervention, particularly through structured group-based activities. Initially, the participant exhibited strong attachment to a single hydrotherapist and hesitated to engage with peers. Over time, he demonstrated increased social flexibility, participating in cooperative swimming games, peer-led challenges, and spatial orientation tasks such as "Follow the Sound," indicating progress in the subdimension of Group cooperation within the Social Belonging and Inclusion dimension. These activities facilitated interaction despite profound visual impairment and encouraged reciprocal communication and teamwork.

Such peer-supported environments have been shown to promote participation and emotional well-being among children with disabilities, particularly in inclusive aquatic settings where differences in physical ability are less visually pronounced (Lambeck & Gamper, 2011). The aquatic space, by minimising hierarchical visual cues, provided a levelled playing field for social connection, reinforcing a sense of belonging and shared achievement.

Given his initial difficulty adapting to unfamiliar facilitators, continued efforts to rotate therapists and integrate peer modelling may further strengthen his social confidence and reduce dependency on specific individuals.

Additionally, systemic supports such as the use of a mechanical hoist, temperature-regulated water, and predictable sensory conditions (e.g., controlled lighting and sound) played a crucial role in advancing the subdimension of Equality, by removing physical and perceptual barriers to participation. Fostering peer-based support also aligns with broader inclusive education and rehabilitation goals, promoting equity and shared agency within therapeutic environments.

Holistic Well-Being and Long-Term Impact

The final dimension of the Four-Dimensional Model considers the sustainability and life-wide integration of therapeutic gains. Although this child had participated in hydrotherapy since infancy, the structured Halliwick programme introduced a progression toward greater autonomy and endurance, supporting the establishment of swimming as a long-term recreational and therapeutic activity.

Importantly, sustained participation requires appropriate environmental and programmatic supports. Due to the risk of exacerbated spasticity in cool water, community-based swimming was recommended only in facilities that maintain therapeutic water temperatures. This environmental consideration is critical to ensuring safe and effective engagement (Becker, 2009; Lambeck & Gamper, 2011). A structured transition plan, including supervised adaptive swimming sessions, peer-supported aquatic exercise, and gradual reduction in therapist support, was proposed to maintain continuity and motivation. These supports aim to reinforce the subdimension of Health behaviour sustainability by promoting lifelong engagement in physical activity, reducing the risk of isolation, and supporting quality of life over time.

While improvements in propulsion, postural control, and social participation were evident, some limitations remained. The participant continued to show caution when navigating novel aquatic settings and experienced fatigue during extended activity. These findings suggest the need for ongoing endurance training, exposure to varied pool environments, and gradual skill generalisation to promote confidence across contexts.

Overall, this case report illustrates the potential of a Halliwick-based hydrotherapy programme to support functional ability, emotional growth, and social integration in a child with severe motor and sensory challenges. By using the Four-Dimensional Model of Hydrotherapy as an analytic lens, the intervention is understood not only as a clinical success but also as a process of empowerment, inclusion, and sustainable engagement in meaningful activity.

Conclusion

This case report demonstrates the value of a Halliwick-based hydrotherapy intervention in promoting mobility, self-efficacy, and social inclusion in a young person with quadriplegic cerebral palsy and cortical visual impairment. By applying the Four-Dimensional Model of Hydrotherapy, the intervention was evaluated not solely in terms of biomechanical improvement, but also across the broader domains of sensory experience, affirmative identity, social belonging, and long-term participation.

Meaningful gains were observed in aquatic mobility, postural control, and the participant's willingness to engage with peers and a wider range of therapists. These improvements reflect not only enhanced functional capacity, but also increased confidence, adaptability, and motivation to engage in water-based activities. Nonetheless, the persistence of anxiety in unfamiliar settings highlights the importance of gradual transition planning and sustained environmental supports to ensure ongoing participation.

This case underscores the relevance of structured, multidimensional aquatic programmes in supporting children with complex neuromotor and sensory profiles. Future research is warranted to explore the long-term sustainability of hydrotherapy-based interventions, particularly in relation to community integration, emotional resilience, and quality of life.

Participant Perspective[11]

When I first started hydrotherapy, I was quite anxious about movement in water. Even though I had been attending sessions since infancy, I still felt uncertain and dependent on my therapist to guide me. I was particularly uneasy when something in my routine changed, such as when my usual therapist was absent. In those cases, I often refused to participate altogether because I felt out of control.

At the beginning of this program, I needed constant hands-on support. Every movement was guided, and I relied entirely on my therapist's instructions. But over time, I started to gain confidence in moving independently. At first, I practiced small, controlled movements, like shifting my weight in the water, but after a few weeks, I was able to propel myself short distances without assistance. That was a huge achievement for me.

One of the activities I found both exciting and challenging was the "Follow the Sound" game, where I had to navigate toward a peer's voice in the water. This was particularly helpful for me, as I have cortical visual impairment, and relying on sound helped me develop spatial awareness and directional control. However, when more people were involved, it became harder for me to distinguish where to move. I think this type of activity would work better with a smaller group or more structured turns, so that it remains effective for participants with visual impairments.

By the end of the program, I felt truly free in the water. On land, I need my wheelchair for everything and rely on others for support. But in the pool, I could move on my own, even if just for a few meters. This gave me a new sense of independence and confidence.

Now, I feel less fearful of movement and more motivated to continue swimming. At first, hydrotherapy was just another therapy I had to do, but now I see it as something I enjoy and want to get better at. I still need warm water to prevent my muscles from stiffening, and I know there are challenges to practicing in larger groups, but I also know I have the ability to move independently, and that's a huge step forward for me.[12]

CHAPTER SUMMARY

The case reports presented in this chapter highlight the multidimensional impact of hydrotherapy, underscoring the value of a holistic framework that extends beyond conventional biomechanical rehabilitation. Each example illustrates the unique yet interrelated dimensions of the Four-Dimensional Model of Hydrotherapy: Body Functioning and Sensory Experience, Affirmative Identity and Self-Determination, Social Belonging and Inclusion, and Holistic Well-Being and Long-Term Impact, demonstrating how these domains manifest across varied clinical contexts.

Together, these cases illustrate that effective hydrotherapy must address not only physical objectives but also the psychological, emotional, and social dimensions of each individual's lived experience. The interventions described reflect the importance of person-centred care, therapeutic alliance, and the transformative potential of water-based rehabilitation in fostering confidence, autonomy, and meaningful inclusion. These case reports contribute not only to clinical practice but also serve as valuable pedagogical tools for students, supervisors, and researchers seeking to implement inclusive, person-centred approaches within aquatic therapy.

As the field of hydrotherapy continues to evolve, it is essential that practitioners are equipped through comprehensive education that integrates clinical expertise with inclusive and interdisciplinary values. The next chapter explores the current landscape of hydrotherapy training, examining how professional preparation can align with the Four-Dimensional Model to support the delivery of meaningful, equitable, and sustainable interventions.

NOTES

1 While the CARE guidelines use the term 'patient' this case report adopts person-centred and inclusive language by referring to the individual as a participant in a therapeutic process.
2 Although the CARE guidelines use the term 'Clinical Findings' this case report adopts an inclusive, person-centred alternative.
3 While the CARE guidelines use the term 'patient' this case report adopts person-centred and inclusive language by referring to the individual as a participant in a therapeutic process.
4 Written informed consent was obtained from the individual for the inclusion of this case report and personal account in this publication.
5 While the CARE guidelines use the term 'patient' this case report adopts person-centred and inclusive language by referring to the individual as a participant in a therapeutic process.
6 Although the CARE guidelines use the term 'Clinical Findings' this case report adopts an inclusive, person-centred alternative.
7 While the CARE guidelines use the term 'patient' this case report adopts person-centred and inclusive language by referring to the individual as a participant in a therapeutic process.
8 Written informed consent was obtained from the individual for the inclusion of this case report and accompanying personal perspective.
9 While the CARE guidelines use the term 'patient' this case report adopts person-centred and inclusive language by referring to the individual as a participant in a therapeutic process.
10 Although the CARE guidelines use the term 'Clinical Findings' this case report adopts an inclusive, person-centred alternative.
11 While the CARE guidelines use the term 'patient' this case report adopts person-centred and inclusive language by referring to the individual as a participant in a therapeutic process.
12 Written informed consent was obtained from the participant and their parent/legal guardian for the publication of this case report and accompanying personal perspective.

REFERENCES

Amras, A., & Kamalakannan, R. (2023). Role of aquatic therapy in knee rehabilitation: A narrative review. *Indian Journal of Physiotherapy and Occupational Therapy*, *17*(4), 1–6.

Becker, B. E. (2009). Aquatic therapy: scientific foundations and clinical rehabilitation applications. *PM&R*, *1*(9), 859–872.

Buckthorpe, M., Pirotti, E., & Della Villa, F. (2019). Benefits and use of aquatic therapy during rehabilitation after ACL reconstruction-a clinical commentary. *International Journal of Sports Physical Therapy*, *14*(6), 978.

Flanigan, D. C., Everhart, J. S., Pedroza, A., Smith, T., & Kaeding, C. C. (2013). Fear of reinjury (kinesiophobia) and persistent knee symptoms are common factors for lack of return to sport after anterior cruciate ligament reconstruction. *Arthroscopy: The Journal of Arthroscopic & Related Surgery*, *29*(8), 1322–1329.

Franco, M. R., Morelhão, P. K., de Carvalho, A., & Pinto, R. Z. (2017). Aquatic exercise for the treatment of hip and knee osteoarthritis. *Physical Therapy*, *97*(7), 693–697.

Gagnier, J. J., Kienle, G., Altman, D. G., Moher, D., Sox, H., & Riley, D. (2013). The CARE guidelines: Consensus-based clinical case reporting guideline development. *Global Advances in Health and Medicine*, *2*(5), 38–43.

Gajić, D., Jokić, S., & Mraković, B. (2020). Efficiency of the Halliwick concept in the rehabilitation of children with cerebral palsy. *Scripta Medica*, *51*(3), 174–180.

Hajouj, E., Hadian, M. R., Mir, S. M., Talebian, S., & Ghazi, S. (2021). Effects of innovative aquatic proprioceptive training on knee proprioception in athletes with anterior cruciate ligament reconstruction: A randomized controlled trial. *Archives of Bone and Joint Surgery*, *9*(5), 519.

Hinman, R. S., Heywood, S. E., & Day, A. R. (2007). Aquatic Physical Therapy for Hip and Knee Osteoarthritis: Results of a Single-Blind Randomized Controlled Trial. *Phys Ther*, *87*, 32–43.

Kurt, E. E., Büyükturan, B., Büyükturan, Ö., Erdem, H. R., & Tuncay, F. (2018). Effects of Ai Chi on balance, quality of life, functional mobility, and motor impairment in patients with Parkinson's disease. *Disability and Rehabilitation*, *40*(7), 791–797.

Lambeck, J., & Bommer, A. (2010). Ai Chi®: Applications in clinical practice. In *Comprehensive Aquatic Therapy* (3rd edn). Washington State University Publishing.

Lambeck, J., & Gamper, U. N. (2011). The Halliwick concept. In J. Lambeck & U. Gamper (eds), *Comprehensive Aquatic Therapy* (3rd edn). Washington State University Publishing.

Little, C., Lavender, A. P., Starcevich, C., Mesagno, C., Mitchell, T., Whiteley, R., Bakhshayesh, H., & Beales, D. (2023). Understanding fear after an anterior cruciate ligament injury: A qualitative thematic analysis using the common-sense model. *International Journal of Environmental Research and Public Health*, *20*(4), 2920.

Martínez-Rodríguez, A., Cuestas-Calero, B. J., García-De Frutos, J. M., & Marcos-Pardo, P. J. (2021). Psychological effects of motivational aquatic resistance interval training and nutritional education in older women. *Healthcare* (Basel, Switzerland), *9*(12), 1665–1665.

McAvoy, R. (2009). Research report: Aquatic and land-based therapy vs. land therapy on the outcome of total knee arthroplasty: A pilot randomized clinical trial. *Journal of Aquatic Physical Therapy*, *17*(1), 8–15.

Mohapatra, M., Rath, S., Agarwal, P., Singh, A., Singh, R., Sutar, S., Sahu, A., Maan, V., & Ganesh, S. (2022). Cerebral visual impairment in children: Multicentric study determining the causes, associated neurological and ocular findings, and risk factors for severe vision impairment. *Indian Journal of Ophthalmology*, *70*(12), 4410–4415.

Nissim, M., Livny, A., Barmatz, C., Tsarfaty, G., Berner, Y., Sacher, Y., Bodini, R., & Ratzon, N. Z. (2021). Effects of Ai Chi practice on balance and left cerebellar activation during high working memory load task in older people: A controlled pilot trial. *International Journal of Environmental Research and Public Health*, *18*(23), 12756. https://doi.org/10.3390/ijerph182312756

Ohji, S., Aizawa, J., Hirohata, K., Mitomo, S., Ohmi, T., Jinno, T., Koga, H., & Yagishita, K. (2021). Athletic identity and sport commitment in athletes after anterior cruciate ligament reconstruction who have returned to sports at their pre-injury level of competition. *BMC Sports Science, Medicine and Rehabilitation*, *13*, 1–7.

Peng, M. (2023). Aquatic exercises in the knee injury rehabilitation of athletes. *Revista Brasileira de Medicina do Esporte*, *29*, e2022_0495.

Pérez-de la Cruz, S. (2020). Influence of an aquatic therapy program on perceived pain, stress, and quality of life in chronic stroke patients: A randomized trial. *International Journal of Environmental Research and Public Health*, *17*(13), 4796.

Prins, J., & Cutner, D. (1999). Aquatic therapy in the rehabilitation of athletic injuries. *Clinics in Sports Medicine*, *18*(2), 447–461.

Riley, D. S., Barber, M. S., Kienle, G. S., Aronson, J. K., von Schoen-Angerer, T., Tugwell, P., Kiene, H., Helfand, M., Altman, D. G., Sox, H., Werthmann, P. G., Moher, D., Rison, R. A., Shamseer, L., Koch, C. A., Sun, G. H., Hanaway, P., Sudak, N. L., Kaszkin-Bettag, M., Carpenter, J. E., & Gagnier, J. J. (2017). CARE guidelines for case reports: Explanation and elaboration document. *Journal of Clinical Epidemiology*, *89*, 218–235.

Rosenblatt, Y., Athwal, G. S., & Faber, K. J. (2008). Current recommendations for the treatment of radial head fractures. *Orthopedic Clinics of North America*, *39*(2), 173–185.

Sokal, P. A., Norris, R., Maddox, T. W., & Oldershaw, R. A. (2022). The diagnostic accuracy of clinical tests for anterior cruciate ligament tears are comparable but the Lachman test has been previously overestimated: A systematic review and meta-analysis. *Knee Surgery, Sports Traumatology, Arthroscopy*, *30*(10), 3287–3303.

Song, J. A., & Oh, J. W. (2022). Effects of aquatic exercises for patients with osteoarthritis: Systematic review with meta-analysis. *Healthcare*, *10*(3), 560.

Viswanath, M., Jha, R., Gambhirao, A. D., Kurup, A., Badal, S., Kohli, S., Parvathi Parappil, P., John, B. M., Adhikari, K. M., Kovilapu, U. B., & Sondhi, V. (2023). Comorbidities in children with cerebral palsy: A single-centre cross-sectional hospital-based study from India. *BMJ Open*, *13*(7), e072365.

Vova, J. A. (2022). Cerebral palsy: An overview of etiology, types and comorbidities. *OBM Neurobiology*, *6*(2), 1–25.

Woby, S. R., Roach, N. K., Urmston, M., & Watson, P. J. (2005). Psychometric properties of the TSK-11: A shortened version of the Tampa Scale for Kinesiophobia. *Pain*, *117*(1–2), 137–144.

Xiang, A., Fu, Y., Wang, C., Huang, D., Qi, J., Zhao, R., Wu, L., Fan, C., & Zhang, Q. (2024). Aquatic therapy for spastic cerebral palsy: A scoping review. *European Journal of Medical Research*, *29*(1), 569–575.

Zaffagnini, S., Grassi, A., Serra, M., & Marcacci, M. (2015). Return to sport after ACL reconstruction: How, when, and why? A narrative review of current evidence. *Joints*, *3*(1), 25.

Zhang, L., Liu, G., Han, B., Wang, Z., Yan, Y., Ma, J., & Wei, P. (2020). Knee joint biomechanics in physiological conditions and how pathologies can affect it: a systematic review. *Applied Bionics and Biomechanics*, *2020*(1), 7451683.

Chapter 7
Future Directions in Hydrotherapy Practice

Hydrotherapy, situated at the intersection of clinical rehabilitation, education, and embodied human experience, must continue to evolve in response to the complex and shifting needs of diverse populations. The Four-Dimensional Model of Hydrotherapy, as outlined in this volume, provides not only a robust conceptual foundation but also a practical framework for guiding future developments in practice, training, and policy. This chapter outlines key strategic directions for embedding inclusive, person-centred, and identity-affirming approaches into the expanding field of aquatic therapy, ensuring that hydrotherapy remains relevant, responsive, and transformative in the years to come.

INTERDISCIPLINARY TEAMWORK

The future of hydrotherapy depends not only on innovative techniques or individual expertise, but on the capacity of professionals to collaborate meaningfully across disciplines. Interdisciplinary teamwork, defined as the coordinated effort of two or more professionals from different fields working towards a shared therapeutic goal, has become essential in addressing the complex and multifaceted needs of individuals with disabilities (Fleming & Monda-Amaya, 2001; Patel, Pratt & Patel, 2008).

Interprofessional collaboration has been conceptualised as a dynamic process grounded in shared goals, mutual respect, and interdependency between professionals, rather than autonomous parallel work. It requires a shift from competition to cooperation and recognition of each discipline's unique contribution (D'Amour et al., 2005). In hydrotherapy, this collaboration brings together aquatic therapists, physiotherapists, occupational therapists, speech and language therapists, nurses, educators, and social workers to design integrated care pathways that reflect the biopsychosocial realities of participants.

DOI: 10.4324/9781003659709-11

Effective interdisciplinary teams are grounded in shared values, trust, and a collective vision. They operate not through hierarchical structures but through cooperative, egalitarian relationships in which each member's expertise is acknowledged and respected. This spirit of equality ensures that challenges faced by one team member are understood as collective concerns, fostering a deep sense of shared responsibility and cohesion.

Although interdisciplinary collaboration is widely advocated as essential for holistic care, robust evidence of its consistent effectiveness remains limited. A comprehensive Cochrane review found that practice-based interprofessional interventions, such as team rounds, facilitated meetings, and shared checklists, may moderately improve functional outcomes and adherence to clinical guidelines. However, the overall certainty of the evidence was rated as low due to methodological inconsistencies, variability in interventions, and limited reporting on team dynamics (Reeves et al., 2017).

Embedding intentional teamwork strategies, grounded in both evidence and professional reflection, can strengthen the integration of physical, emotional, and social goals in hydrotherapy. Interdisciplinary teamwork is shaped by dynamic processes of communication and reflection. Information sharing involves each professional bringing specialised knowledge about the participant, contributing their unique perspective, and aligning progress goals. Consultation emerges through reflective dialogue in which team members explore clinical dilemmas and co-construct therapeutic strategies.

Organisational structures and formalised processes play a vital role: clearly defined leadership roles, regular interdisciplinary meetings, time allocated for joint planning, and a shared vision that reflects the values of inclusive, person-centred care. Without these supports, collaboration tends to remain superficial or revert to siloed practices (Sicotte et al., 2002).

Professionals may be socialised within discipline-based frameworks that can hinder mutual understanding. Interprofessional collaboration therefore requires resocialisation and the development of shared cognitive and value maps (Clark, 1997; D'Amour et al., 2005). Creating a culture of openness and curiosity is essential for surfacing tensions and transforming them into opportunities for dialogue, boundary negotiation, and collaborative resolution. Informal interpersonal conversations, structured reflection, and real-time observation during therapeutic practice can all offer valuable insights into team dynamics. Ongoing facilitation, provided by supervisors, trainers, or peer mentors, can support the development of high-functioning teams and prevent breakdowns in communication (Brownell et al., 2006).

Despite growing policy emphasis on coordinated, interdisciplinary service provision, implementation in practice remains inconsistent and fragmented. A UK qualitative study on Education, Health and Care (EHC) plans for children and young people with disabilities highlighted significant challenges in achieving effective collaboration across sectors. Families often reported a lack of communication, delayed planning processes, and confusion regarding professional responsibilities (Adams et al., 2018).

The integration of participants themselves into aspects of team reflection and planning, whether through formal feedback processes or participatory goal-setting – remains underdeveloped in many contexts Recent research highlights ongoing barriers to eliciting the voices of children with disabilities in such planning processes (Sharma, 2021). Yet this practice is increasingly recognised as essential for achieving meaningful and ethical outcomes (D'Amour et al., 2005).

Competencies for interdisciplinary teamwork, such as openness to feedback, respectful engagement with difference, and shared decision-making, should be integrated early in professional education. Hydrotherapy programmes should incorporate interprofessional modules, experiential learning, and opportunities for reflection on power, communication, and collaboration. For experienced practitioners, ongoing training and structured opportunities for peer dialogue remain essential.

Interdisciplinary teamwork in hydrotherapy is not simply an operational model, but a foundation for ethical, inclusive, and effective care. When supported through intentional structures, shared values, and evidence-informed practices, teamwork enables more responsive interventions, stronger professional relationships, and better outcomes for participants. Above all, it reflects a shift from isolated care to collective growth, among professionals, and with the individuals they support.

Viewed through the lens of the Four-Dimensional Model of Hydrotherapy, interdisciplinary teamwork enhances each of the model's core dimensions. Collaborative clinical planning enriches the Body Functioning and Sensory Experience dimension by allowing professionals to integrate physical, cognitive, and sensory knowledge into unified interventions. Through respectful dialogue and shared reflection, teamwork supports Affirmative Identity and Self-Determination, as professionals co-construct therapeutic environments that honour participants' agency and preferences. The very structure of teamwork, rooted in shared responsibility and mutual support, mirrors the aims of Social Belonging and Inclusion, creating not only inclusive care plans but inclusive working cultures. Finally, interdisciplinary collaboration contributes to Holistic Well-Being and Long-Term Impact by ensuring continuity of care, psychosocial sensitivity, and sustained progress across therapeutic domains. In this way, teamwork becomes not only a professional ideal, but a conduit through which inclusive, person-centred rehabilitation is brought to life.

TRANSFORMATIVE EDUCATION

Reimagining hydrotherapy education in the 21st century requires more than technical updates to existing curricula. It calls for a deep pedagogical shift, a transformation in how practitioners are prepared to understand disability, engage with diversity, and deliver person-centred care. This shift finds its theoretical grounding in the framework of transformative learning, as conceptualised by Mezirow (1997), who argued that adult education should enable individuals to critically examine, and ultimately revise, their frames of reference through processes of reflection, dialogue, and emancipatory learning.

In this view, learning is not merely the acquisition of skills or knowledge, but a fundamental reorientation of meaning structures: the values, assumptions, and expectations through which professionals interpret their work, relationships, and responsibilities. Such transformation is essential for hydrotherapy practitioners. Mezirow's distinction between instrumental and communicative learning is particularly relevant. While instrumental learning focuses on task efficiency and technical competence, communicative learning aims to foster understanding of meaning, context, and human complexity (Mezirow, 1997). Hydrotherapy education has historically prioritised the former, with its emphasis on biomechanical principles, safety protocols, and method-based instruction. However, inclusive and rights-based practice necessitates a shift towards the latter, enabling practitioners to explore the social, emotional, and cultural dimensions of disability and care.

Building on Mezirow's theory, contemporary research highlights how transformative learning processes unfold in clinical education. A recent scoping review found that learners who experience disorienting dilemmas, such as confronting personal biases, encountering unfamiliar perspectives, or facing ethical uncertainty, are more likely to engage in critical self-reflection and undergo meaningful professional growth (Vipler et al., 2021). These findings support the integration of transformative pedagogies into hydrotherapy training, particularly through methods such as narrative-based learning, structured reflection, critical incidents analysis, and community-based placements.

In parallel, reflective practice plays a central role in facilitating this transformation. Reflection not only deepens learning but also supports identity development and professional reasoning (Mann et al., 2009). In the hydrotherapy context, reflection enables students and practitioners to process emotional responses to close physical contact, to examine implicit assumptions about disability, and to develop relational attunement. These reflective habits of mind are essential for ethical and inclusive decision-making in the complex, fluid, and intimate space of the therapeutic pool.

To create the conditions for transformative learning, hydrotherapy education must intentionally embed experiences that challenge assumptions, provoke dialogue, and invite reflexivity. The Four-Dimensional Model introduced in this book provides a framework for doing so. By structuring training around bodily functioning and sensory experience; affirmative identity and self-determination; social belonging and inclusion; and holistic well-being and long-term impact, the model encourages learners to move beyond mechanistic approaches and toward care that is relational, contextual, and socially aware.

Practical strategies to support this pedagogical shift include simulation exercises that explore communication with non-verbal participants, such as using symbol-based communication boards in the pool environment. Reflective journaling may be used to explore emotional responses to physical proximity, dependency, or discomfort, for example, following an aquatic session with a participant who has undergone limb amputation. Programmes may also incorporate co-teaching with disability activists or peer mentors, enabling learners to engage directly with the lived experiences and perspectives of those they support. Finally, community-based placements in inclusive aquatic or recreational settings allow students to contextualise hydrotherapy within everyday life, rather than solely within pool frames. These methods do not merely transmit knowledge; they actively shape how learners perceive themselves and others, as therapists, collaborators, and agents of inclusion.

Importantly, transformative education is not a one-time event, but a lifelong process. Continuing professional development for hydrotherapists should include opportunities to revisit and re-examine their assumptions, engage with evolving disability discourse, and reflect on practice through interdisciplinary supervision and peer dialogue. Without such opportunities, even well-trained practitioners risk falling back into task-oriented or paternalistic habits.

Although the direct correlation between transformative learning and improved service outcomes remains a developing area of research, the literature consistently supports its role in fostering professional competence, empathy, and ethical awareness (Mezirow, 1997; Mann et al., 2009; Vipler et al., 2021). In the case of hydrotherapy, where the therapeutic relationship is embodied, immersive, and deeply human, such education is not simply beneficial, it is imperative.

In line with scholarship that repositions continuing professional development within the realities of professional practice (Boud & Hager, 2012), future directions in hydrotherapy education must also attend to the evolving needs of experienced practitioners. Beyond formal courses and credit-based learning, ongoing development should be embedded within the practice itself, through peer mentorship, interdisciplinary exchange, reflective dialogues, and cross-contextual learning opportunities. Such approaches reframe professional learning not as the passive acquisition of knowledge but as a dynamic process of participation, construction, and becoming. When framed through the Four-Dimensional Model, this invites not only students but also seasoned professionals to re-engage with their identities, values, and social commitments, ensuring hydrotherapy remains a living, growing field grounded in critical inquiry and inclusive care.

Transformative hydrotherapy education must not only equip practitioners to deliver inclusive care, but also ensure that learning environments are themselves inclusive of diverse learners and educators, including individuals with disabilities. When the principles of the Four-Dimensional Model are applied to education, Body Functioning and Sensory Experience invites curriculum designers to consider sensory needs, physical access, and multimodal engagement. Affirmative Identity and Self-Determination becomes relevant not just to clients but to learners and lecturers, particularly those with disabilities, who must see their identities affirmed, their autonomy respected, and their contributions valued within professional education. Social Belonging and Inclusion calls for pedagogical communities where disabled and non-disabled students, supervisors, and academic staff collaborate, co-teach, and co-create knowledge. And Holistic Well-Being and Long-Term Impact reminds us that education is not only a pathway to qualification but to meaningful participation, long-term confidence, and future leadership. By centring the lived experiences of all participants in the learning process, transformative education realises its full emancipatory potential, not only shaping better therapists, but cultivating more equitable and diverse systems of care and knowledge production.

In sum, reconceptualising professional education in hydrotherapy through the lens of transformative learning enables the development of practitioners who are not only clinically competent, but also critically reflective, socially attuned, and committed to equity. By engaging with learners as whole people, cognitively, emotionally, and ethically, education becomes a space not only for acquiring technique, but for forming the professional identities and values that underpin truly inclusive care.

INCLUSIVE ORGANISATIONAL CULTURE

Embedding inclusion within the organisational culture of hydrotherapy services requires more than policy declarations or isolated practices. It involves a deep reconfiguration of the values, structures, and routines that shape how care is delivered, how teams function, and how people with disabilities are perceived and involved. Inclusion must also be viewed through the lens of human rights and legal frameworks, as emphasised in European disability law (López-Sáez, 2015).

To move towards this vision, organisations must first interrogate their own assumptions about disability and difference. Even institutions that outwardly claim to support inclusion often reproduce exclusionary dynamics through hidden curricula, disciplinary hierarchies, or narrow definitions of professionalism (Morley & Croft, 2011). Inclusive organisational cultures challenge these patterns by prioritising voice, agency, and relationality, particularly for those who have historically been marginalised within care systems. This includes not only clients, but also professionals with disabilities and those from culturally and linguistically diverse backgrounds. Co-produced interventions, such as those involving neurodiverse children and their families, illustrate how redistributing power and designing with rather than for participants can foster mutual trust and relevance (Armitt et al., 2024).

The Equipping Primary Health Care for Equity (EQUIP) framework offers a powerful model for integrating equity-oriented approaches into health service delivery (Browne et al., 2015). It emphasises trauma- and violence-informed care, cultural safety, and harm reduction, not only as clinical competencies, but as organisational commitments. Applied to hydrotherapy, this model invites services to consider how therapeutic environments, team dynamics, and institutional policies can either reinforce or challenge existing inequities. For example, promoting shared decision-making, ensuring accessibility of spaces and communication, and actively involving participants in programme design are all structural expressions of inclusion.

Organisational leadership plays a pivotal role in cultivating inclusive cultures. Without clear commitment from senior staff and service managers, even the most dedicated practitioners may struggle to implement inclusive approaches. This includes allocating time and resources for interdisciplinary meetings, reflective supervision, and co-production with service users. As highlighted in the literature on disability education, superficial interventions are unlikely to bring about lasting change (Shakespeare & Kleine, 2013); sustained engagement, supported by policy and structure, is essential. Sustainable inclusion relies not only on values but also on the operationalisation of inclusive dialogue, documentation, interpretation, and understanding within organisational routines. Recent work highlights these mechanisms as essential to achieving engagement and alignment in participatory service design (Masterson et al., 2024).

Leadership must also take responsibility for challenging systemic health inequities faced by people with disabilities. Despite increasing policy commitments, individuals with disabilities continue to experience worse health outcomes and significant barriers to care, resulting in dramatically shortened life expectancy in many contexts (Kuper et al., 2025). Leadership in hydrotherapy and rehabilitation services must therefore address not only inclusion in theory but also equity in practice, through accessible design, responsive policy, and advocacy for systemic reform.

Importantly, embedding inclusion also means rethinking who counts as a 'knower' or an 'expert' within therapeutic systems. When people with disabilities are positioned as co-educators, co-designers, or advisors, they help shift the culture from one of charity or compliance to one of partnership and justice. The recognition of individuals with disabilities as agents of knowledge is essential to countering tokenism and enabling meaningful participation (Morley & Croft, 2011).

Finally, inclusive cultures are built through everyday interactions. Language, tone, touch, and listening are not neutral; they carry cultural and relational significance. Staff training must therefore include not only technical knowledge but also critical reflection on power, embodiment, and social difference. This is echoed in the EQUIP framework's emphasis on ongoing reflexivity and the cultivation of environments where both staff and participants feel safe to express vulnerability and complexity (Browne et al., 2015).

Creating an inclusive organisational culture also requires the cultivation of reflective capacity across all levels of the workforce. Reflection, defined as the deliberate examination of values, assumptions, and experiences in order to achieve deeper understanding, is increasingly recognised as essential for ethical and person-centred practice (Mann et al., 2009). Reflective practice is not simply an individual trait, but a shared organisational competency that must be nurtured through ongoing dialogue, mentorship, and learning environments that legitimise vulnerability and complexity. Research suggests that professionals develop deeper reflective capacity when supported by emotionally safe environments, inclusive leadership, and opportunities for collaborative reflection, factors that mirror those required for inclusive care delivery itself (Mann et al., 2009). Embedding structured reflective opportunities into supervision, team meetings, and organisational routines can help align day-to-day interactions with the values of justice, humility, and partnership that underpin inclusive hydrotherapy.

Embedding inclusion into organisational culture is a transformative, ongoing process. It calls for alignment between values and practice, between leadership and frontline work, and between the organisation and the communities it serves. For hydrotherapy to truly fulfil its holistic promise, inclusion must be lived, not only in theory, but in every policy, posture, and practice. In sum, an inclusive organisational culture is not a peripheral feature but a structural foundation for ethical, person-centred hydrotherapy. When inclusion is embedded in policies, leadership, daily interactions, and reflective practice, it transforms services from sites of care delivery into spaces of empowerment, belonging, and shared growth. Rooted in the values of the Four-Dimensional Model, such cultures affirm the worth of every participant, clients, staff, and collaborators alike, and ensure that diversity is not simply acknowledged, but meaningfully woven into the fabric of professional life.

INCLUSIVE INFRASTRUCTURE, TECHNOLOGY, AND ACCESS

Despite the growing recognition of hydrotherapy's benefits, multiple barriers continue to limit equitable access to aquatic rehabilitation (Carlsson et al., 2022). These include physical, financial, cultural, and infrastructural constraints, each of which must be addressed through design, adaptive strategies, and forward-thinking policy. Embedding accessibility into hydrotherapy is not only a matter of ethics, but of practical innovation and sustainability.

Accessibility barriers continue to affect many aquatic facilities (Yeomans et al., 2024). Accessibility audits of public aquatic spaces, including swimming pools, showers, and saunas, have identified mobility-related barriers that may limit participation for individuals with disabilities, unless inclusive and adaptive infrastructure is implemented (Carlsson et al., 2022). Inadequate features such as the absence of pool hoists, ramps, or accessible changing areas frequently hinder equitable engagement. Recent findings from a study involving students with disabilities at the University of British Columbia further reveal that challenges extend beyond the built environment, encompassing limited staff training and poorly designed spatial layouts. For example, excessively steep ramps, inaccessible washrooms, and staff discomfort or lack of confidence in providing appropriate support can discourage participation and pose safety concerns (Godfrey et al., 2024). In addition, sensory accessibility remains an often-overlooked yet critical component. Overcrowding, loud music, harsh lighting, and unwelcoming social atmospheres can create sensory overload. These highlight the importance of sensory-sensitive adaptations, such as quiet hours, softer lighting, and clearer signage, alongside respectful staff communication and an inclusive, welcoming facility culture (Godfrey et al., 2024).

According to the World Report on Disability, inaccessible infrastructure, including transport systems, public buildings, and aquatic facilities, remains a significant barrier to full participation for individuals with disabilities. The report emphasises that ensuring access to mainstream environments should not be treated as a supplementary effort, but as a core obligation within rights-based frameworks (Officer & Posarac, 2011). This perspective is echoed by Imrie (2012), who critiques approaches to universal design that prioritise technical fixes over structural change, arguing that accessibility must be embedded as a principle of justice rather than a market-based accommodation. In the context of hydrotherapy, this reinforces the necessity for inclusive design from the outset, not as a reactive retrofit, but as a foundational commitment to equity and participation.

Globally, standards such as the Americans with Disabilities Act (ADA) (United States, 1990) offer a framework for improving accessibility and should inform design and retrofitting of hydrotherapy environments.

Financial barriers also restrict participation (Godfrey et al., 2024), especially in underserved or rural communities where pool construction and maintenance are prohibitively expensive. Public-private partnerships, mobile pools, and subsidised community-based aquatic programmes have demonstrated success in expanding access, particularly when guided by local needs and cultural relevance.

A promising example of resource-sensitive, community-based hydrotherapy can be found in a recent feasibility study which examined a cross-sector intervention for individuals with musculoskeletal conditions (Wilson et al., 2024). The programme was delivered through a partnership involving National Health Service (NHS) physiotherapy services, a local leisure centre, and a social enterprise specialising in AI-guided aquatic rehabilitation. This collaborative model demonstrates how limited resources can be navigated through creative design, public-health alignment, and social innovation. By leveraging existing community infrastructure, such as municipal swimming pools, the programme reduced the need for dedicated facilities, making it more scalable and adaptable across settings. The use of waterproof tablets offering individually tailored aquatic exercise routines, developed by the social enterprise Good Boost, enabled a high degree of personalisation while minimising therapist time. In this way, hydrotherapy was anchored within existing networks of health, leisure, and voluntary services, turning everyday community environments into therapeutic spaces. The model also incorporated trained volunteers who supported participants during sessions, combining clinical benefit with social connection. Volunteer engagement enhanced cost-effectiveness and fostered intergenerational inclusion, reinforcing the Social Belonging and Inclusion and Holistic Well-Being and Long-Term Impact dimensions of the Four-Dimensional Model of Hydrotherapy.

In terms of financial accessibility, the programme adopted a progressive pricing structure, offering an initial free session followed by low-cost participation. This approach balanced sustainability with equity and could be adapted to diverse national contexts through partnerships between health insurers, municipal services, and local Non-Governmental Organizations (NGO). Finally, structured peer support was integrated as a key component, with participants engaging in group-based activity followed by informal social interactions, such as shared refreshments. These moments of social exchange not only increased motivation and adherence, but created a sense of community ownership and psychological safety, elements often overlooked in facility-based care.

Together, these features illustrate how hydrotherapy services can be reimagined through inclusive, participatory, and contextually embedded approaches. Rather than viewing limited budgets or infrastructure as insurmountable barriers, this model exemplifies how collaboration and creativity can extend the reach and impact of aquatic rehabilitation in equitable and sustainable ways.

Cultural and psychological barriers must not be overlooked. Fear of water, cultural discomfort with shared swimming spaces, or lack of information about hydrotherapy's benefits can all hinder engagement. Addressing these challenges requires culturally sensitive outreach, water confidence initiatives, and the co-creation of services with community stakeholders to foster trust and inclusion.

To reduce fear and build water confidence, gradual, small-group sessions led by trained instructors can be effective. In culturally diverse communities, offering gender-specific sessions and permitting culturally appropriate swimwear may enhance comfort and participation. Such accommodations respect cultural norms and encourage individuals who might otherwise feel uncomfortable in mixed-gender settings.

Collaborating with local leaders and community health workers as 'hydrotherapy ambassadors' can bridge gaps in understanding and increase trust in the intervention. These ambassadors can effectively communicate the benefits of hydrotherapy and address specific community concerns, fostering a supportive environment for participants. Family-inclusive programming, such as intergenerational sessions may increase motivation. Collectively, these strategies may not only improve attendance and emotional safety but also reinforce the dimensions of Social Belonging and Inclusion and Holistic Well-Being and Long-Term Impact within the Four-Dimensional Model of Hydrotherapy.

In addition, hydrotherapy must also evolve in response to environmentaland infrastructural constraints. In many regions, limited access to aquatic facilities, whether due to space shortages, seasonal climate fluctuations, or water scarcity, can significantly restrict service availability. To ensure continuity and equity of care, creative and sustainable adaptations are essential.

Creative adaptations have begun to emerge in response to environmental and facility constraints. For example, circuit-based programming enables small or shared pools to accommodate multiple participants efficiently by rotating between stations or time slots, thus maximising spatial use while ensuring safety and therapeutic value (Buckthorpe et al., 2019). Such approaches are especially relevant in resource-limited or high-demand settings.

In regions where climate poses limitations, mobile pools with solar-heated systems have been trialled as flexible, energy-efficient alternatives, enabling outreach in underserved or remote communities. While specific peer-reviewed studies on mobile hydrotherapy pools remain scarce, related research and documented implementations support the feasibility of such systems. For example, ur Rehman, Hirvonen, and Sirén (2017) analysed several configurations of community-scale solar heating systems in cold climates. Their findings demonstrated that combinations of solar thermal collectors with seasonal borehole storage and heat pumps can provide up to 81% renewable energy coverage for heating needs, even in high-latitude settings. These technologies offer adaptable models for thermal management in off-grid or remote areas, suggesting applicability for mobile aquatic settings that require sustainable heat sources. Additionally, a large-scale case study conducted in Dade County, Florida demonstrated the economic and operational feasibility of using solar-heated systems in public swimming pools. The initiative not only extended the annual usability of the pool but also achieved substantial cost savings and increased community engagement. The system relied on unglazed polypropylene panels and basic local infrastructure, making it a replicable model for low-resource settings. The project further illustrates the potential for community-driven, solar-powered aquatic programmes to be implemented sustainably at the municipal level (Levin, 1981).

Together, these sources offer a compelling basis for envisioning solar-heated mobile hydrotherapy units as viable innovations, especially where conventional infrastructure is constrained by climate, geography, or funding.

The use of natural water bodies, such as lakes, rivers, or geothermally heated springs, offers a promising and ecologically grounded approach to expanding hydrotherapy access, particularly in regions where built infrastructure is limited. When accompanied by appropriate safety protocols, trained staff, and environmental oversight, these settings can serve as effective therapeutic environments. Beyond their practicality, nature-based solutions have been shown to enhance the sensory and emotional dimensions of therapy. Research on open-water swimming highlights benefits such as reduced psychological distress, increased emotional regulation, and strengthened social bonds, particularly through immersion in so-called 'blue spaces' (Overbury et al., 2023). A large-scale international study further found that swimming in natural environments, compared to artificial pools, was associated with greater improvements in mental well-being, largely due to the sense of autonomy, competence, and connection fostered by natural settings (Groeneveld et al., 2025). These findings suggest that, when implemented inclusively and safely, nature-based hydrotherapy can support not only physical rehabilitation but also holistic well-being and long-term psychological resilience.

Such innovations not only broaden the geographical reach of hydrotherapy but also align with ecological values and local resource availability. When embedded within community-led planning, these adaptations have the potential to create inclusive, resilient, and context-sensitive hydrotherapy programmes that thrive even in resource-constrained settings.

Technological innovation is a key driver of future accessibility. Emerging tools such as waterproof wearable sensors, virtual reality (VR), and smart pool systems offer new ways to tailor interventions, enhance engagement, and track progress in real time. VR, for example, enables immersive, gamified movement scenarios that improve motor control, motivation, and psychological readiness, particularly among individuals recovering from neurological or musculoskeletal conditions. A growing body of research supports the therapeutic benefits of VR in aquatic settings. For instance, a recent randomised controlled trial by Saleh and Abozed (2024) demonstrated that children undergoing hydrotherapy for burn injuries who received VR intervention experienced significantly lower pain levels, more stable physiological parameters, and faster wound healing compared to a control group receiving standard care. These findings underscore the role of VR not only as a distraction tool but as a clinical adjunct that enhances both physical and emotional rehabilitation outcomes. This is consistent with broader reviews of clinical VR, which highlight its role in improving pain tolerance, attention, and emotional regulation in complex rehabilitation scenarios (Rizzo et al., 2017). Smart pools equipped with underwater cameras and resistance calibration systems further allow therapists to customise interventions with precision and provide real-time feedback to participants. In addition to rehabilitation-focused technologies, recent advancements in artificial intelligence (AI) and the Internet of Things (IoT) are reshaping how aquatic environments are monitored for safety. A review describes next-generation drowning prevention systems that integrate embedded sensors, computer vision, and real-time alert technologies to detect unsafe situations swiftly and accurately (Kao et al., 2024). This integration of AI and IoT within smart pool environments offering an added layer of protection and autonomy that aligns with principles of inclusive design and equitable access to hydrotherapy.

In parallel, wearable technologies are increasingly being utilised to monitor underwater movement patterns and physiological responses. A systematic review identified 27 studies employing inertial measurement units (IMU) and other waterproof sensors to assess aquatic exercise, highlighting promising applications in capturing joint angles, muscle activity, and spatial orientation (Monoli et al., 2023). Kos and Umek (2018) developed a sensor-based system for aquatic rehabilitation that utilises a waterproof IMU placed on the swimmer's lower back. Their model enables real-time feedback on stroke symmetry, roll angle, and fatigue detection, offering therapists clinically meaningful insights during aquatic sessions. The authors propose three complementary modes of application, therapist-guided, autonomous, and cloud-based, thereby supporting both immediate intervention and longitudinal progress tracking. This wearable solution illustrates the potential of sensor-based hydrotherapy to enhance therapeutic precision while empowering participants through data-driven personalisation. Beyond its clinical precision, this approach offering participants greater autonomy and engagement regardless of physical ability or communication style. In this way, wearable technologies can play a critical role in access to responsive and person-centred hydrotherapy.

Ultimately, these approaches do more than enhance access, they model a shift towards hydrotherapy as a fully integrated component of community health, inclusion, and lifelong well-being. As we look to the future, it is imperative that hydrotherapy not only evolves through innovation but remains grounded in the principles of inclusivity, community engagement, and lived experience. Accessibility must be reconceptualised not as a retroactive accommodation, but as a fundamental design element in hydrotherapy research, education, and practice.

REFERENCES

Adams, L., Tindle, A., Basran, S., Dobie, S., Thomson, D., Robinson, D., & Codina, G. (2018). Education, health and care plans: A qualitative investigation into service user experiences of the planning process. Department for Education. https://repository.derby.ac.uk/download/0050f1414f9dbb4d345d2dbcd06911147a5b40ca035878b8b9bda92ac15f034a/902082/2018_Education_Health_and_Care_plans_-_a_qualitative_investigation.pdf

Armitt, H. A., Attwell, L., Kingsley, E. N., White, P. C., Woolley, K., Garside, M., Green, N., & Coventry, P. A. (2024). Reflections and practical tips from co-producing an intervention with neurodiverse children, their families, and professional stakeholders. *Humanities and Social Sciences Communications*, *11*(1), 1–11.

Boud, D., & Hager, P. (2012). Re-thinking continuing professional development through changing metaphors and location in professional practices. *Studies in Continuing Education*, *34*(1), 17–30.

Browne, A. J., Varcoe, C., Ford-Gilboe, M., Wathen, C. N., & EQUIP Research Team. (2015). EQUIP Healthcare: An overview of a multi-component intervention to enhance equity-oriented care in primary health care settings. *International Journal for Equity in Health*, *14*, 1–11.

Brownell, M. T., Adams, A., Sindelar, P., Waldron, N., & Vanhover, S. (2006). Learning from collaboration: The role of teacher qualities. *Exceptional Children*, *72*(2), 169–185.

Buckthorpe, M., Pirotti, E., & Della Villa, F. (2019). Benefits and use of aquatic therapy during rehabilitation after ACL reconstruction-a clinical commentary. *International Journal of Sports Physical Therapy*, *14*(6), 978.

Carlsson, G., Slaug, B., Schmidt, S. M., Norin, L., Ronchi, E., & Gefenaite, G. (2022). A scoping review of public building accessibility. *Disability and Health Journal*, *15*(2), 101227.

Clark, P. G. (1997). Values in health care professional socialization: Implications for geriatric education in interdisciplinary teamwork. *The Gerontologist*, *37*(4), 441–451.

D'Amour, D., Ferrada-Videla, M., San Martin Rodriguez, L., & Beaulieu, M. D. (2005). The conceptual basis for interprofessional collaboration: Core concepts and theoretical frameworks. *Journal of Interprofessional Care*, *19*(sup1), 116–131.

Fleming, J. L., & Monda-Amaya, L. E. (2001). Process variables critical for team effectiveness: A Delphi study of wraparound team members. *Remedial and Special Education*, *22*(3), 158–171.

Godfrey, E., Au, R., Ramos, V., Chan, A., Carino, C., & Zhou, A. (2024). Accessibility Considerations for Choosing a Fitness Centre: Perspectives from UBC Students with Disabilities.

Groeneveld, W., Krainz, M., White, M. P., Heske, A., Elliott, L. R., Bratman, G. N., Lora E. Fleming, L. E., Grellier, J., McDougall, C. W., Nieuwenhuijsen, M., Ojala, A., Pahl, S., Roiko, A., van den Bosch M., & Wheeler, B. W. (2025). The psychological benefits of open-water (wild) swimming: Exploring a self-determination approach using a 19-country sample. *Journal of Environmental Psychology*, *102*, 102558.

Imrie, R. (2012). Universalism, universal design and equitable access to the built environment. *Disability and Rehabilitation*, *34*(10), 873–882.

Kao, W. C., Fan, Y. L., Hsu, F. R., Shen, C. Y., & Liao, L. D. (2024). Next-Generation swimming pool drowning prevention strategy integrating AI and IoT technologies. *Heliyon*, *10*(18).

Kos, A., & Umek, A. (2018). Wearable sensor devices for prevention and rehabilitation in health-care: Swimming exercise with real-time therapist feedback. *IEEE Internet of Things Journal*, *6*(2), 1331–1341.

Kuper, H., Mpanju-Shumbusho, W., & Shakespeare, T. (2025). Building leadership in disability inclusion in health. *The Lancet*.

Levin, M. (1981). Solar-heated municipal swimming pools, a case study: Dade County, Florida (No. SSEC/SP-32266). Southern Solar Energy Center Planning Project, Atlanta, GA (USA).

López-Sáez, M. M. (2015). Social inclusion of persons with disabilities as a human rights issue: new developments and challenges under European Law. *Revista europea de derechos fundamentales*, (26), 193–217.

Mann, K., Gordon, J., & MacLeod, A. (2009). Reflection and reflective practice in health professions education: a systematic review. *Advances in Health Sciences Education*, *14*, 595–621.

Masterson, D., Lindenfalk, B., Kjellström, S., Robert, G., & Ockander, M. (2024). Mechanisms for co-designing and co-producing health and social care: a realist synthesis. *Research Involvement and Engagement*, *10*(1), 103.

Mezirow, J. (1997). Transformative learning: Theory to practice. *New Directions for Adult and Continuing Education*, *1997*(74), 5–12.

Monoli, C., Tuhtan, J. A., Piccinini, L., & Galli, M. (2023). Wearable technologies for monitoring aquatic exercises: A systematic review. *Clinical Rehabilitation*, *37*(6), 791–807.

Morley, L., & Croft, A. (2011). Agency and advocacy: Disabled students in higher education in Ghana and Tanzania. *Research in Comparative and International Education*, *6*(4), 383–399.

Officer, A., & Posarac, A. (2011). *World Report on Disability*. Geneva, Switzerland: World Health Organization.

Overbury, K., Conroy, B. W., & Marks, E. (2023). Swimming in nature: A scoping review of the mental health and wellbeing benefits of open water swimming. *Journal of Environmental Psychology*, *90*, 102073.

Patel, D. R., Pratt, H. D., & Patel, N. D. (2008). Team processes and team care for children with developmental disabilities. *Pediatric Clinics of North America*, *55*(6), 1375–1390.

Reeves, S., Pelone, F., Harrison, R., Goldman, J., & Zwarenstein, M. (2017). Interprofessional collaboration to improve professional practice and healthcare outcomes (Review). *Cochrane Database of Systematic Reviews*, *2017*(6), Article CD000072.

Rizzo, A., & Koenig, S. T. (2017). Is clinical virtual reality ready for primetime? *Neuropsychology*, *31*(8), 877.

Saleh, S. E. S., & Abozed, H. W. (2024). Technology and Children's health: Effect of virtual reality on pain and clinical outcomes during hydrotherapy for children with burns. *Journal of Pediatric Nursing*, *78*, e155–e166.

Shakespeare, T., & Kleine, I. (2013). Educating health professionals about disability: a review of interventions. *Health and Social Care Education*, *2*(2), 20–37.

Sharma, P. (2021). Barriers faced when eliciting the voice of children and young people with special educational needs and disabilities for their education, health and care plans and annual reviews. *British Journal of Special Education*, *48*(4), 455–476.

Sicotte, C., D'Amour, D., & Moreault, M. P. (2002). Interdisciplinary collaboration within Quebec community health care centres. *Social Science & Medicine*, *55*(6), 991–1003.

United States. (1990). *Americans with Disabilities Act of 1990, 42 U.S.C. § 12101 et seq*. Available at: www.ada.gov/

ur Rehman, H., Hirvonen, J., & Sirén, K. (2017). A long-term performance analysis of three different configurations for community-sized solar heating systems in high latitudes. *Renewable Energy*, *113*, 479–493.

Vipler, B., Knehans, A., Rausa, D., Haidet, P., & McCall-Hosenfeld, J. (2021). Transformative learning in graduate medical education: a scoping review. *Journal of Graduate Medical Education*, *13*(6), 801–814.

Wilson, N., Barcellona, M., Lambert, P., Storey, P., Foster, B., Waller, B., & Wilkins, B. (2024). Feasibility of a community-based aquatic and peer support intervention for people with musculoskeletal disorders delivered via a cross-sector partnership: A service evaluation. *Musculoskeletal Care*, *22*(4), e1950.

Yeomans, C., Storr, R., Sherry, E., & Karg, A. (2024). Social value accumulation through Australian aquatic facilities. *Managing Sport and Leisure*, 1–16.

Afterword

Hydrotherapy is more than a therapeutic technique, it is a transformative space where individuals experience recovery, empowerment, identity formation, and social connection. Throughout this book, I have explored the evolution of hydrotherapy from its medicalised origins into a dynamic, inclusive, and person-centred field. The Four-Dimensional Model of Hydrotherapy offers a holistic framework that integrates physical function, affirmative identity, social belonging, and long-term well-being, recognising hydrotherapy as a practice where individuals do not simply recover, they thrive.

Looking ahead, the future of hydrotherapy lies in its capacity to adapt, technologically, socially, and ethically. At the same time, expanding access to hydrotherapy remains a critical goal.

The Four-Dimensional Model places inclusivity and lived experience at its core. This model not only reframes hydrotherapy around individual strengths and autonomy, but also offers a shared language that supports collaboration between therapists, educators, policy-makers, and individuals engaging in aquatic therapy. It recognises that movement is not only biomechanical, it is personal, emotional, social, and meaningful.

Moving forward, this field must continue to grow through interdisciplinary collaboration, inclusive education, and research that captures the full spectrum of hydrotherapy's impact. Training programmes grounded in the Four-Dimensional Model can prepare practitioners to deliver care that honours each individual's narrative, identity, and goals. Policy-makers are also called upon to integrate hydrotherapy into public health, education, and community planning, viewing it not as an alternative therapy, but as an essential, evidence-based component of lifelong well-being.

DOI: 10.4324/9781003659709-12

This book is not a conclusion, it is a beginning. The discourse surrounding hydrotherapy must remain open, intersectional, and guided by those with lived experience. As we integrate technological tools, promote social equity, and embrace affirmative models of disability, hydrotherapy has the potential to become not only more effective, but more just.

To hydrotherapy practitioners, may you centre empowerment, belonging, and holistic outcomes in your work.

To educators and trainers, may you use this framework to prepare future generations with compassion, rigour, and creativity.

To researchers, may you continue expanding the evidence base in ways that capture not just physical outcomes, but emotional and social transformation.

And to those who engage in hydrotherapy firsthand, your experience is the heart of this field. Your voice must shape where it goes next.

Hydrotherapy is not merely a treatment. It is a practice of resilience. A place of safety. A celebration of movement in all its forms.

May it continue to evolve, as a discipline, a community, and a space for equity, affirmation, and hope.

Index

Note: Information in tables is indicated by page numbers in **bold**.

For Product Safety Concerns and Information please contact our EU
representative GPSR@taylorandfrancis.com
Taylor & Francis Verlag GmbH, Kaufingerstraße 24, 80331 München, Germany